ON LAUGHTER-
SILVERED WINGS

ON LAUGHTER-
SILVERED WINGS

by ROBERT E. JACKSON JR., MD

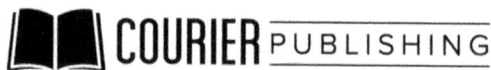

COURIER PUBLISHING

Greenville, South Carolina

CourierPublishing.com

PRINTED IN THE UNITED STATES OF AMERICA

DEDICATED TO

Abbot Land Jackson Carnes

The best mom I ever had
To which she always says,
"I am the *only* mom you ever had."

TABLE OF CONTENTS

INTRODUCTION

In the writing of this book, I have learned much about my parents and their extended families that I did not know. The many conversations with family and friends were such a delight as they shared their memories of my dad, his brothers and sisters, and their parents. During my research and conversations, the topic often veered toward Abbot, my amazing mom, and the high esteem in which she is held. To hear them bragging on her delighted me to no end.

I smiled frequently, laughed aloud occasionally, and wept unashamedly while writing Dad's biography. As you read, I hope you will laugh out loud and realize the appropriateness of the title, since humor and laughter were such a big part of Dad's life. You will smile, you will laugh, and, no doubt, you will weep with me.

Just for clarity — I refer to myself as Robin throughout the book, which is the nickname my mother gave me at birth so I would not be known as "Little Robert." I couldn't escape being "Little Doc," but I did escape being called "Little Robert." When I went to Clemson, my professors called me "Robert" — my designation on their computer printouts. I grew weary of correcting them with "My name is Robin." I eventually gave up — so everyone at Clemson, medical school, and residency knew me as Robert. I ended up with a dual identity. If friends from college and med school asked friends from Manning, "Oh, you're from Manning, so do you know Robert Jackson?" each one would respond, "No, I don't think so." If my Manning friends asked my friends in the Upstate, "Oh, you're from the Upstate, so do you know Robin Jackson?" they would respond, "No, we don't think so." I'm convinced I could commit a terrible crime and just blame it on the other guy, and no one would be the wiser! (Just kidding!) Now you understand why I, the author, am named "Robert" but refer to myself as "Robin" throughout most of the book. It also helps to call me Robin to delineate between my dad and me.

I also go back and forth calling my father Robert, Dad, Captain Jackson, or Dr. Jackson. One name or another just seemed more appropriate in certain places.

High Flight

By John Gillespie Magee Jr.

(An American pilot killed December 11, 1941, at the age of nineteen
during a training flight in Britain. Magee flew with a Spitfire squadron
with the Royal Canadian Air Force during World War II.)

Oh! I have slipped the surly bonds of earth
And danced the skies on laughter-silvered wings;
Sunward I've climbed, and joined the tumbling mirth
Of sun-split clouds — and done a hundred things
You have not dreamed of — wheeled and soared and swung
High in the sunlit silence. Hov'ring there,
I've chased the shouting wind along, and flung
My eager craft through footless halls of air …
Up, up the long, delirious burning blue
I've topped the wind-swept heights with easy grace
Where never lark or ever eagle flew —
And, while with silent, lifting mind I've trod
The high untrespassed sanctity of space,
Put out my hand, and touched the face of God.

When I was in high school, Dad and I often stayed up late to watch the sign-off at midnight on one of the three available television stations during the 1970s. We did it for one reason and one reason only — to hear Dad's favorite poem "High Flight" read by a deep, baritone voice while a jet airplane soared through the deep, blue stratosphere. Dad was a private pilot, and I was a pilot-in-training. The reading was inspirational and thought-provoking as we pondered the possibility of hurling our "eager craft through footless halls of air" and ultimately touching "the face of God." After the screen eventually turned to snow and static, we both slowly turned to each other and shared a deeply satisfying smile. Every time I hear the poem "High Flight," or I spontaneously quote part of it to myself, I recall the fondness of this oft-repeated ritual between my father and me.

On Laughter-Silvered Wings is the long-overdue story of my dad's life. Characterized by great joy in living, his life overflowed with laughter and mirth — both a part of his everyday existence. No doubt he could be profoundly serious at times, even intimidating — but I'm convinced he possessed the "joy of the Lord" as his strength. Making people laugh was a part of his daily routine, both as a physician and friend to many. After all, "a merry heart doeth good like a medicine" (Proverbs 17:22, KJV).

Flying high — yes, flying higher than most of those around him — symbolically describes his life. Driven to strive for excellence in academics and athletics during his youth — and then later in medicine, aviation, the shooting sports, and in civic duties as an adult — he could never rest. He pushed himself to perfect his art and skill in every area of his life. Consequently, he "slipped the surly bonds of earth" and ascended to the "windswept heights" in his every endeavor, becoming a leader in just about every arena of his life. (Except for singing — I'm pretty sure he paid my way through college with the money my church paid him for not singing in the choir.)

Like the author of "High Flight," he "flung his eager craft through footless halls of air" and did "a hundred things you've not dreamed of."

My dad flung himself eagerly at life and accomplished, as one friend said, "more in forty-one short years than most do in an entire lifetime." Although his story ends with a mixture of sadness, yet Christian hope, I'm convinced you will enjoy reading about his journey as he danced his way through life "on laughter-silvered wings," until at last, indeed, he "put out [his] hand and touched the face of God."

ON LAUGHTER-
SILVERED WINGS

1

Doc, I'm Hit

Suddenly, the unmistakable crack of a rifle shot rang out. The sergeant staggered back two steps, clutching his chest, and gasped, "Oh, Doc, I'm hit." He fell backwards off his deck onto a small patch of grass. Captain Jackson stepped away from the operating table, quickly appraised the situation, and vaulted the railing of the porch surrounding the hospital. He caught the sergeant under his arms as he staggered across the yard while yelling, "Somebody shot me." With the assistance of his medic, Bob Kosha, they eased the sergeant onto a stretcher and into the operating room. A quick assessment revealed an entrance wound on the left mid-back under the scapula, and a large exit wound on the anterior left shoulder. The exit wound poured blood, and a loud sucking sound emitted with each inspiration.

♦　♦　♦　♦　♦

The windows of the heavens opened, and the late season monsoon deluged the earth with a flood reminiscent of Noah's experience. Averaging around thirty-eight inches of rain, the rainy season in the mountainous portion of northern Laos would linger for another month before closing out, thus ending the "summer monsoon." As the ever-present clouds lifted from the mountaintops, the daily afternoon downpours would eventually lessen in frequency and intensity. In the lowlands, workers cared for the flooded rice paddies on every plain where green shoots of new growth began to emerge. Conversely, in the mountains, the people planted dry rice seed on every patch of open ground they could find on the steep mountainsides. Eking out a living on the mountains was much more laborious, much less productive.

The clay airstrip in Sam Thong would soon dry out — allowing planes and helicopters to land with less difficulty, bringing supplies and wounded soldiers as the warfare increased during the dry season. Thus, the dry season meant more death and destruction throughout Southeast Asia, including northern Laos, where the American CIA fought a secret war against the North Vietnamese — secret, because the American military had no official presence there. Nevertheless, the undercover effort was desperately needed to support the indigenous American allies and stem the rising tide of Communism in the region.

Private American contractors under the employ of the CIA, the United States Agency for International Development (USAID), Air America, and several other organizations/businesses worked in Laos. Some were considered paramilitary advisors, some worked at the embassy, and some served for charitable reasons; then there were military men who divested themselves of any official affiliation with the American military. In 1966, one such volunteer was Captain Robert E. Jackson, a physician from the 101st Tactical Air Commando Wing. Stationed in Sam Thong — the USAID refugee operations center and a mountain village 100 miles north of Vientiane, the capital of Laos — Captain Jackson posed as just another employee working alongside Dr. Khammoung (also called Dr. K.), a Laotian surgeon trained in France. An outside observer at that time might conclude Jackson's role was as a missionary doctor or perhaps a USAID employee, but his actual status was intentionally murky. With the benefit of declassified documents, it is now apparent that he was actually employed by the CIA.

Captain Jackson networked closely with pilots employed by Continental Air Transport (CAT) and Air America, an airline secretly owned by the United States government but connected to the CIA. His primary mission was to assist in the rescue and care of downed American airmen. Any American pilot in distress over North Vietnam was instructed to try to escape to Laotian territory, where friendly forces could assist in their rescue. Rescued and injured pilots were airlifted to Sam Thong, where there was a dirt airstrip and a rudimentary hospital. Dr. Jackson's second responsibility was to promote humanitarian and goodwill efforts among the mountain people of northern Laos.

"So, Don, how did you come to be in Sam Thong?" The interrogator was Captain Jackson. His accent was southern but not slow. He spoke in short, clipped sentences that seemed to accentuate his words in such a way that one tended to remember his exact words for a long time. He stared at his subject through dark, bushy eyebrows with piercing, hazel eyes that seemed to lock in to the conversation, but at the same time observe all of the activity around him. His directness and the intensity of his focus gave his listeners the distinct impression that he was fully aware of all his surroundings, and he knew exactly where he was going. Men with true leadership capabilities always have a clear vision of their objectives in life and know exactly how they intend to get there. The captain was such a man, and others followed him willingly. Despite his assertiveness, his friends felt comfortable in his presence and sensed a void in his absence. His hair cut short in military fashion, he was clothed in a green scrub suit and had recently left the operating room after a busy day of surgery with Dr. K.

Captain Jackson and Don Scott, a Christian missionary, sat on the bamboo porch of the 100-bed hospital, which was raised three feet off the ground to avoid the mud of the rainy season and to provide a breeze in the hot, dry season. The previous night's rain still dripped from the eaves.

Don responded, "Doc, I'm here because God called me to this place. I first heard about the need for missionaries here in 1958 when I heard a missionary speaker from Laos in our church. I was in the Canadian Navy at that time, but I felt so moved by the challenge to work with the Hmong people that I never forgot the sense of God's call upon my life to prepare for missionary service when I got out of the Navy. It really is a miracle that I'm even here."

"What was the miracle, Don?"

"Well, I was honorably discharged early from the Navy due to serious eczema on my hands that hindered my work. I had suffered eczema from early childhood. It would clear up and then return from time to time. When I applied for overseas service along with Nola [Don's wife], my lifelong problem with eczema came up, of course, and I had to have a dermatologist's assessment of it. I truly expected to be denied the opportunity to serve."

"Yet here you are."

"Yes, by the grace of God! I went to see the required specialist, and upon my arrival at his office, I had no trace of eczema anywhere on my body! My hands were completely normal, although just days before they were covered with eczema blisters. The doctor was totally surprised because he had seen my records. He concluded that I would be more useful to the mission overseas than I would be a detriment and recommended me for service where the climate is cooler and the food's not so spicy! So here we are! Nola and I arrived with a six-month-old daughter not too long ago. So, Doc, how about you? Why are you in Laos?"

After a long pause, gazing at the surrounding mountains that reminded him of the Blue Ridge Mountains back home in South Carolina, the captain responded, "My military friends told me I was crazy to come up north in Laos, but I volunteered. I was bored to tears handling sick calls in the dispensary back at Udorn. Didn't even know what the mission fully entailed. I was just told it was of great importance to the war effort, and it would be dangerous, so I volunteered." Pausing only for a moment, he then added, "My time here has been some of the most interesting and challenging of my entire life!" Then he resumed staring out at the distant mountains surrounding Sam Thong with a pensive gaze.

"Do you regret it?" Don asked hesitantly.

The response was immediate. "No, not one instant. I've loved these people like you do. It's strange how God puts a love in my heart for a people that I don't even know or understand. I don't know their language or their culture, but God puts affection in my heart for each one of them. More than that, I love practicing tropical medicine. Do you realize that in the States I never treated malaria, typhoid, or malnutrition like I do here? At home I treat diseases like hypertension, diabetes, and elevated cholesterol, mostly caused by overeating. Here, I treat infectious diseases resulting from poor sanitation and malnutrition, because people do not have enough to eat. I feel like I'm making a difference here that is substantially different than my contribution in the States. The only healthcare these Laotians have is the local witch doctor, which is essentially no healthcare at all. More than that, the wounded soldiers and civilians would die if not for the urgent care provided by Dr. K. and myself. No, I don't regret volunteering. The humanitarian work here is desperately needed. The goodwill established will pay dividends for America for generations to come."

With that, he jumped to his feet and bounded across the muddy expanse to the OR, kicking his knees up high in that peculiar fashion of his, as if he were walking through a "freshly plowed field." He always seemed to be in a hurry, always on a mission, ready to change the world.

Six hours and four surgeries later (one appendectomy, one inguinal hernia, debridement of a shrapnel wound in the arm, and amputation of a lower extremity injured by a North Vietnamese booby trap), Dr. Jackson scrubbed up after surgery, fatigued but pleased with the day's accomplishments. Even in the rainy season, they performed four or five surgeries per day — removing goiters, repairing hernias, removing abdominal tumors, and repairing hand and foot injuries caused by land mines or the ever-present booby traps that injured women and children as well as the soldiers. Of course, during the dry season, soldiers with bullet or shrapnel wounds came through their hospital almost daily, brought in by airlift or carried on pallets by their fellow soldiers. The war surrounded Sam Thong. Most assuredly, it was not a safe place.

While Dr. Jackson and Dr. K. proceeded to operate on a patient's badly injured knee, their X-ray tech, a US Army sergeant, sauntered outside of the operating room to gaze at the city of Sam Thong — a city of 20,000 people situated in a valley surrounded by mountains 6,000 feet in height. Walking over to his living quarters, he sat on his deck to read a book. Suddenly, the unmistakable crack of a rifle shot rang out. The sergeant staggered back two steps clutching his chest and gasped, "Oh, Doc, I'm hit." He fell backwards off his deck onto a small patch of grass. Captain Jackson stepped away from the operating table, quickly appraised the situation, and vaulted the railing of the porch surrounding the hospital. He caught the sergeant under his arms as he staggered across the yard while yelling, "Somebody shot me." With the assistance of his medic, Bob Kosha, they eased the sergeant onto a stretcher and into the operating room. A quick assessment revealed an entrance wound on the left mid-back under the scapula, and a large exit wound on the anterior left shoulder. The exit wound poured blood, and a loud sucking sound emitted with each inspiration.

"Quick, hand me two large towels," Dr. Jackson ordered. A Laotian nurse trained by Dr. Jackson and Dr. K. jumped into action, handing him two sterile towels — which were instantly placed over the wounds, front and back. He then grabbed a sterile chest tube from a nearby surgical tray and inserted it deftly into the left chest between the ribs, thereby releasing the tension pneumothorax in his left chest. Approximately 500 cc of blood came pouring out through the newly inserted tube. "All right, start an IV with a large bore needle. I want Lactated Ringers, and run it in as fast as it will go. Get a plane ready. We can't do this type of surgery here." Only five minutes had elapsed since he had been shot, and already he was stabilized with a chest tube and IV fluids. If only wounded soldiers on the field could receive such immediate care!

Dr. K. responded with a look of despair and said, "He'll never make it.

We should try to do something here."

"No, we are not properly equipped. We'll fly him south to Korat Army Hospital in Thailand." At that moment the heavens opened, and the midnight rain fell hard on the tin roof of the OR, drowning out all communication.

Dr. K. shouted, "You'll never be able to take off in this weather."

"Maybe not, but we will try. Get that IV running." Pointing at an orderly, "You go get the pilot ready. Tell him that as soon as there is a break in the weather, we intend to leave."

Dr. K. and the OR staff were stricken. "Captain, we could lose both of you and a pilot. Please reconsider," begged Dr. K.

"I'm not going to risk the pilot's life, but if this rain stops, we will try to get this soldier to a proper OR."

Everyone stared at Dr. Jackson. The patient was sweating and gasping for breath as the good doctor held his hand. "Go get Don," Dr. Jackson requested, staring down at his wounded X-ray tech. "We need him to pray over this soldier and our flight."

Thirty minutes later, as flame pots lined the runway and dark clouds clung to the 6,000-foot surrounding mountains, the rain stopped. The ominous clouds hung at 500 feet over the wet clay runway. Their severely wounded patient and Captain Jackson were already loaded in the back of a single engine U-10. The patient was semi-conscious, his pulse weak and thready, his breathing erratic. Both the pilot and Dr. Jackson were tense but ready. The doctor shouted over the engine's roar, "Fly in a tight circle until we reach 8,000 feet, then fly directly south." Only twenty-two years old, the young but experienced marine pilot nodded grimly and then responded, "Doc, they pay you to care for the wounded. They pay me to fly. Don't you worry a bit." The prop spun faster as the engine revved up; the wheels started rolling, and the small plane lifted off and quickly disappeared into the darkening sky. Using the flame pots as a guide, the U-10 flew in tight circles until reaching 8,000 feet, then flew directly south by dead reckoning since no radio signals were available. Don huddled up with a small group of nurses and Dr. K. on the runway and began to pray, "O, Lord, our Lord, keep them safe …"

Flying through darkness and constant rain squalls, the little Helioplane reached Udorn Air Force Base after an hour of a tension-filled flight. There the patient and his doctor were transferred to a C-130 and transported to Korat AFB, where a more sophisticated OR was available at the Army hospital. Upon arrival at Korat, rather than finding a surgeon and an OR prepared for them, Captain Jackson discovered a psychiatrist on night call "who didn't know his rear end from a hole in the ground" (his thought to himself in a disheartening moment). Already fatigued, the captain had to care for his wounded X-ray tech for several more hours until a surgeon came on duty at 8:00 a.m.

This shooting event occurred about ten days after the nurses at the Sam Thong hospital staged a protest due to dissatisfaction with their pay. It was the jungle version of a labor union protest, just without the labor union. The X-ray tech became indignant, went to the nurses' homes, pulled several of them out of their beds and forced them to go to work. His actions were unacceptable and contrary to the customs of the Laotian people. Americans and other foreigners were not allowed to touch one of the indigenous people, male or female; plus, the tech had absolutely no authority over the nurses. It required several days of strenuous effort on the part of Pop Buell, who operated the USAID program at Sam Thong, to pacify the nurses. Then, subsequent to this event, the foolish X-ray tech was playing around with one of the nurses on the day prior to the shooting in full view of the Laotian soldiers. Captain Jackson had a premonition that his X-ray tech's tenure at the hospital would be abbreviated because of his actions. Indeed, he suspected trouble might be brewing. However, he expected a transfer — not an emergency evacuation!

Finally, Dr. Jackson left his patient and returned to Sam Thong. Upon his arrival, a contingent of Air America pilots greeted the good doctor, receiving him like a newly anointed hero. As they stood in a circle around the tired, smiling doctor, one of them, obviously appointed as the spokesman for the group, said, "Doc, we have all decided that even though we have access to a company doctor, if any of us is wounded in action we want you to take care of us. We have confidence in you. By the way, we all think you should get a medal for what you did for your X-ray tech the other night. That was above and beyond the call of duty!"

Receive a medal he did — the Bronze Star for "meritorious achievement, outstanding medical skill, and courage under extremely hazardous conditions." The captain was up-country for one month, and already he was a hero to the local pilots and nominated for a major military award.

Dr. Jackson's conduct demonstrated the twofold reasons for his presence in the secret war in Laos — to take care of American soldiers and to foster a good relationship between Americans and Laotians. He fully understood his responsibilities and intended to do his dead level best to fulfill them. In a letter home to his wife immediately following the above incident in mid-August 1966, he commented regarding his goodwill efforts, "In every respect, I try to be gracious and polite to the nurses because they are only one step removed from the jungle. They are trying to learn. A friendly smile means a lot to them. The nurses look to me, the doctor, to look out for them. They mean well, even if they do start IVs on the wrong patients!"

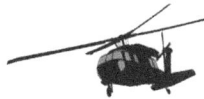

2

HUMBLE BEGINNINGS

In the 1700s, Isaac Jackson moved from White Plains, Virginia, to North Carolina, and then to the Camden District of South Carolina. There he purchased 140 acres on the east side of Nasty Branch, the tributary of Black River in what was then called Claremont County, later part of the Sumter District. Four generations later, Moultrie Reid Jackson (M.R.) was born on a farm in Sumter County in South Carolina. He was the second oldest of eight siblings with five brothers and two sisters. He described his home life as happy and congenial, even though he and his siblings were expected and required to perform a great deal of farm and home labor.

Through a home correspondence course, M.R. learned how to be a telegrapher, which afforded his first employment for the Southern Railroad. He worked for the railroad for a few years, but then returned to the farm at his mother's insistence, since his father had died about six years previously in 1904.

Approximately three years later, he married Anna Charlotte Singleton, also of Sumter County. Her lineage can be traced all the way back to Christopher Singleton, who hailed from the Isle of Wight in England. Christopher left there to settle in Caroline County, Virginia, with his wife, Mary. Christopher's son, Robert, and his wife, Gail, left Virginia in the 1700s to settle in Sumter County.

M.R. farmed on rented land in Sumter until 1924 — at which time, entirely on credit, he purchased a 300-acre farm and house in Clarendon

County in the Sammy Swamp area. The following is a description of the house summarized from *Clarendon Cameos*:

> Constructed around 1835 on the Old Georgetown Road, the M.R. Jackson House (or the Jackson House, as it was fondly called in later years) initially had two large rooms forming the core of the first level of the house. By the time M.R. owned the house, the pegged, heart-of-pine flooring of the original house had long been covered over, but the pegs could be seen from underneath the house. The original structure was built by E.G. "Ellie" DuBose. After his death in 1895, Harmon Timmons acquired the house, which he then rented to Dr. Williams Easterling Dinkins. After Dr. Dinkins' death in 1905, Henry Beatson purchased the house, who enlarged and remodeled it around 1909 by adding an upstairs porch and connecting the kitchen to the house with an open breezeway. Subsequent remodeling removed the upstairs porch and closed in the breezeway, resulting in a simple, modified colonial-style home. At this stage, Moultrie Reid Jackson acquired the house in 1924, and resided there until his death in 1971. The last owner of the house was Carl F. Jackson, the next-to-youngest son of M.R.

The house had fallen into disrepair by the time M.R. purchased it, so he pursued repairs as finances became available — that is, until the Great Depression five years later. Most of the older children were in school by this time, so M.R. decided the oldest sons would run the farming operation while he sought additional employment to support a growing family. In 1933, he obtained a job as a land appraiser with the Federal Land Bank, considerably improving the financial position of the family.

Eunice, one of M.R.'s two daughters, remembered her daddy as a "very reserved and serious man. Mama was the exact opposite of this. We had so much fun with Mama. She had a beautiful soprano voice and often sang solos in church. She didn't get to church very often because of so many small children to care for. When Mama was well, she was such a joy to all of us and we had so much fun together. Sometimes we had biscuit dough fights. We would take a little ball of dough and throw it at each other. At times we would throw it up to the ceiling to try to make it stick up there. Jehu was involved in some of this mischief with us. Mama would laugh until tears streamed down her face. When I was sixteen after I started driving, I took Mama to a baseball game to watch M.R. [Jr.], Jehu, and Billy play ball. Two of the teachers were taking up money from the people in attendance. When we got to the gate, Mama said to them, 'I have three sons playing ball, and I am not going to pay to see the game.' I was mortally embarrassed. The teachers told Mama if they had three sons playing they would not pay either, so we walked right through.

"When we were growing up, our toilet was an outhouse on the west side of our home out in the field. We referred to it as a privy or backhouse. It had a long seat built on one side, which could accommodate five people (two adults and three children) at one sitting — although I don't recall ever having five in there at one time. Our mama was in the outhouse one day when Jimmy and I started throwing clumps of dirt at it. Mama shouted, 'Stop,' and then she said, 'Go get switches off the peach tree for your whipping.' She whipped us good that morning and we learned a good lesson."

I wish I could say September 18, 1936, was a momentous day for the Jackson family, but I kind of doubt it, since the arrival of a new baby was a common occurrence in the Jackson home. That day was my dad's birth day, and, as it turned out, he was the last child born to M.R. and Anna. The parents had run out of names by this time, so the naming of the newest Jackson baby went something like this:

Anna's second son Jehu, along with his friend Edward Broadway, eagerly asked, "What are you going to name this baby?"

His mother replied, "I haven't decided yet."

In unison, they cried out, "Let us name him!"

Anna replied, "Put it on him." Thus, the distinctive name of Robert Edward landed on the last baby after Jehu's friends Robert Thomas and Edward Broadway.

Having experienced mood swings most of her adult life, Robert's mother fell into a deep, dark depression several months after he was born. She had contracted the flu and then progressed into the depression, from which she never recovered. She had premonitions of her early demise for months in advance. After the family doctor, Dr. Harvin, told her husband, M.R., that she needed to go to a hospital in Columbia, Anna handed Robert, now nine months old, to her oldest daughter Eunice, and said, "Sister, take care of my baby. I may not be coming home." Slowly and sadly, she also took off her wedding ring and gave it to Eunice. A month later, on July 15, 1937, Anna, the mother of ten children, went to her reward.

The entire family was shocked and saddened by her death. Eunice and Edna, the two daughters, immediately began to assume the role of mother in the life of the household. Their untiring care and direction were responsible in great measure for the proper upbringing of the younger children.

In the confusion and the despair after Anna's death, the newborn baby boy was taken to the home of a nearby neighbor, Virginia Richards Sauls, a thirty-four-year-old married woman with one child of her own. After keeping Robert for a while, she offered to adopt him since she had been unable to bear another child and to ease the distress of the Jackson family. However, her father, John Gardiner Richards from Liberty Hill, a former governor of South Carolina, spoke words of wisdom to her, saying, "Virginia, you're still of age to bear a child of your own. I recommend that you take that baby boy back to the Jackson family." By then, several weeks had passed, during which she had become emotionally attached to the handsome baby boy. She pondered long and hard her duty to the Jackson family with nine other children and her own desire to have another child.

More than that, when M.R. learned of her interest in adopting his youngest child, he informed her that though the Jackson family was grateful for her help, they were fully capable of taking care of their newborn baby boy. Ultimately, she listened to M.R. and to the advice of her father, who was wise enough to govern an entire state and to speak wisdom into the life of his own daughter. She returned young Robert to the care of his sixteen-year-old sister Eunice. Later, Virginia gave birth to Morgan, who would become best friends with Robert's brother Carl, and John Land, the brother of Robert's future wife.

At age sixteen, Eunice Jackson became the mother figure of four boys all under the age of eight — Ralph, Scott, Carl, and Robert. Years later, Eunice wrote in her personal memoirs:

Afterwards, there was no thought of my going to college. I knew the little boys were my responsibility, and I never felt otherwise.

About a week after Mama passed, I was cleaning up the house. Suddenly, the thought hit me, "Ole girl, you can't be slack anymore. Mama isn't coming behind you. You have to sweep under the beds every day and also do all of the housecleaning."

Two weeks later, the three youngest boys took whooping cough. I rocked babies and cried many days and nights. After recovering, Robert continued to have ailments the entire following winter. He slept with me or in a little cradle beside my bed. He was my baby to care for and Carl was Jimmy's. When he would not sleep and cried, I put him in the cradle and rocked it with my foot. We slept in an upstairs bedroom with no heat. I warmed several bottles each night before going to bed, wrapped them in towels, and put them under my pillow. They stayed warm until he wanted them. Each morning I took him downstairs to the old kitchen, bathed him beside the wood stove, fed him his breakfast, and gave him a teaspoon of cod liver oil to take care of his vitamin needs.

I carried him up and down the stairs. I'd carry him up the stairs in one arm, and I held onto a lamp with the opposite hand. I never dropped the lamp once.

Each summer for many years, Carl and Robert had sore eyes and ground itch. Robert often carried a corn cob in his pocket when he was a little boy to use for scratching between his toes to relieve the itching.

When all of us were growing up, we never had any problems with the boys, not anything. None were unkind to each other nor to me, but Carl and Robert did get teed off at each other some.

Our home was plenty big, but we had too few baths. All of the boys got in the bath at the same time, while I bathed upstairs with a basin of soap and water. We bathed in cool water most of the time, but we occasionally heated water on the stove. We had no electricity. When lights came on for the first time in 1949, it liked to have scared Daddy to death. We had a drop cord in all of the rooms and one receptacle in the dining room, which is where we did all of the ironing.

Our family attended First Baptist Church of Manning, but I don't think Mama went to church much because she stayed home with all of the babies. Daddy would have us at church by 9:00 a.m., even though Sunday School started at 10:00. He would never allow us to be late for anything. He always had to allow time for a flat tire or some other misadventure so he would not be late. He was the Sunday School secretary for many years and also a deacon.

Our father was a quiet, religious man who worked hard every day from before sunrise until dark. He always tried to instill into us the importance of living Christian lives, the importance of honesty, watching the company you keep and paying your debts. Many times, he would lecture to us at night about the necessity for doing better, good behavior, and hard work. One expression we often heard was, "We are turning over a new leaf tomorrow." [I find this rather humorous because I heard my father, Robert, say this to us numerous times. The apple doesn't fall far from the tree.]

The boys worked hard on the farm during the summers. During school days, Daddy got us up before daylight every day. It was very difficult getting up out of bed when the weather was cold and dark, then going downstairs to stand by the fireplace to get dressed. The boys milked the cows and fed the mules and hogs before going to school.

None of the four youngest brothers remembered their real mother. The only mother they ever had was Eunice. Ralph said:

She cared for us after Mama died. She was a tender worker, and she never complained. She washed our clothes, prepared our meals, and got us ready for school. Every Saturday night, she washed all of us in a #2 washtub. She had a real servant's heart — not just when we were young, but all of her life. She would also referee when Scott and I got into a fight, which was just about every day. Most of the time a peach switch was adequate, but once when I was older, Eunice could only find a yard stick, which she promptly broke in two over my backside. She was a big sister, a mama, and a disciplinarian all in one. What a difficult job.

Scott, who was four when his mother died, remembered:

Eunice fed us, clothed us, and kept us straight. She took us to Penny's department store in Sumter once a year right before school started to buy us clothes. She got all four of us dressed and off to school every day. Ralph and I tussled every day. She had to whip us every day — her daily routine. Daddy worked in St. Matthews as a land surveyor Monday through Friday, while Billy worked the farm. Eunice had responsibility for us boys. She had to be the kindest and sweetest person I ever knew. She couldn't have been a better mother.

Carl remembered Eunice as a peacemaker:

Once I had a tricycle that Scott took away from me. I promptly took an air rifle and shot him in the thigh with it. Next thing I knew, we were tussling on the ground in a cloud of dust. Sister Eunice had to settle that dispute. Our daddy kneeled by the bed to pray every night at bedtime. On one occasion, Robert and I had made little bows out of sticks and strings, and arrows out of broom straw from Sister Eunice's broom. While Daddy was kneeling and praying, Robert and I shot broom stick arrows at his backside. Despite this distraction, Daddy just kept right on praying.

Aunt Eunice's son Mike was born when her youngest brother, Robert, was three years and three months old. Mike said:

I was raised with my uncles, but I really thought they were my brothers. We played together, slept together, and fought together. Mama bathed us all together on Saturday nights in the same washtub. Every time she took a peach tree limb to them, I got it, too. We never missed Sunday School or church because of Mama's influence. I remembered even when I was young that she read her Bible continuously. She loved to sew and made clothes for my uncles and eventually her own children. I can truly say that my mama was a saint. I never heard her say a bad word or say anything bad about anyone else.

Robert always called Eunice "Sister." On one occasion, he looked at me and said very seriously, "Son, this is my mother. She raised me." Personally, I had a great deal of affection for my aunt Eunice — not just because she was my aunt nor for the excellent character qualities she possessed, but because she was a mother to my dad. She raised him to be a God-fearing, right-thinking Christian man who, in turn, greatly influenced me in my spiritual pilgrimage.

By 1937, the Depression was beginning to ease, and M.R. Jackson found employment with the Farm Security Administration as assistant county supervisor. The older sons continued operating the farm. In 1940, M.R. was promoted to assistant state tenant purchase specialist for District Three, which was comprised of seven counties. Delighted to serve in that capacity, he helped tenant farmers become owners of their farms and homes. Having come from such humble beginnings himself, he gladly helped other farmers become private property owners. During this time, he was able to pay off the mortgage on the Jackson farm, and, for the first time, enjoy being debt-free.

With the help of his sons, M.R. continued to farm during the years leading up to and during World War II. His farming operation grew cotton, tobacco, corn and small grain for sale — and raised cattle, hogs and chickens for consumption by the family. The Jackson farm produced yields equal to the best in the county by keeping abreast of the best farming methods. He utilized Agrico Fertilizer and Pedigreed Seed exclusively after 1954. His farm often won the Five Acre Cotton Contest and was a member of the 100 Bushel Corn Club. A great-grandson commented, "You can't get more southern than that!"

At the county fair every year, local farmers showed their best produce, cows, or hogs. One year, M.R. had a large photo of all his children placed above his produce. Extremely proud of his ten children and their accomplishments, he placed a caption under the photo that read, "My best crop ever!"

All ten children graduated from Manning High School. The boys participated in all forms of athletics during their high school years. When Robert,
the youngest, finished in 1954, the Lions Club of Manning in a public
ceremony presented M.R. with a football with the names of the boys and
the years they played on the team inscribed on it. The oldest son, Moultrie
Reid, began playing in 1930, and the youngest, Robert, finished in 1954.

Five of the boys (four graduated) attended Clemson College (now
Clemson University), and one, Scott, played on the football team, making
the varsity squad his freshman year. He made ACC All Conference and
during his fourth year was named the Most Valuable Player on the team.

Through the years, M.R. Jackson participated in various civic activities. For a number of years, he served on the board of trustees for the
local school and gave much time to organizing the local county fair. He
also served on the board of deacons of Manning First Baptist Church and
was the general secretary of the Sunday School for twenty years. It was
his habit to read through his Bible and John Milton's *Paradise Lost* once
per year. He occasionally met to compare notes with Ms. Nina McFadden,
who lived down the road at Live Oak, to share what each of them had
been learning from their studies. He was truly a lifelong learner. One of
the charter members of the county Farm Bureau, he served ten years as its
president, receiving multiple recognitions and awards for his service.

My first cousin Johanna, only two years younger than her uncle Robert
as the daughter of Robert's older brother Billy, recalled:

Papa Jackson was known for his desire to be punctual. He
often said, "If you can't get there early, don't bother to go." Papa
Jackson always had a household rule that the entire family should
be present at the breakfast table before anyone could begin eating.
I recall the time when I spent the night at Papa's house, and I tried
to sleep in the next morning. Papa made all of the boys sit at the
breakfast table, staring at heaping platters of steaming eggs and

fried bacon while he stood at the bottom of the stairs and hollered, "Johanna, Johanna, you better hurry down to breakfast. These boys are hungry and waiting on you." I could not believe that Robert, Carl nor Scott had warned me in advance.

In his last years, Papa Jackson drove a blue Rambler pickup, and despite declining health and failing memory, he continued to inspect the immense fields of corn and tobacco being raised by his sons — a far cry from the 300 acres he once operated.

He always kept a hoe in the back of his truck. Despite his sons owning the newest and latest equipment for cultivating huge corn fields, he would crawl out of that blue Rambler and grab his hoe if he saw any weeds in the field. With a handle blackened by years of use and a metal blade worn down to an inch and a half by years of hard hoeing, he would start hoeing at one end of a long row and then disappear into the shadows cast by corn stalks much taller than he, not stopping until he chopped every weed. It wasn't unusual for a family member to drive by and see his blue Rambler truck parked by the roadside, but no sign of Papa — because he would be lost in hundreds of acres of corn. The entire family had to be called out to walk the corn rows to find Granddaddy Jackson — or Papa Jackson, as he was variously called. Most times he would be found, safe and sound, busily hacking away at unwanted weeds. However, on one occasion the family found him prostrate from a stroke in the middle of a very large corn field. He was sternly warned by his youngest son, the doctor, not to ever do such a thing again, but the farmer in him could not stop. Ultimately, his hoe and his blue Rambler had to be confiscated by Robert, the family doctor. What a sad day!

M.R. went to be with Jesus in 1971 at the age of eighty-two, surrounded by all his children and more than thirty grandchildren. A few years later, on August 3, 1978, much to the sorrow of friends, family and really to all of those who knew and appreciated its history, a fire totally destroyed the iconic "M.R. Jackson" home. Flames leaping hundreds of feet in the night sky could be seen from several miles away. About fifty spectators gathered to watch the demise of the old home place, a Clarendon County landmark for almost 150 years. For years afterwards, whenever I drove by the charred remains of the "Old Jackson Homeplace," I couldn't help but become emotional as I recalled all the family reunions and Sunday afternoon picnics held on the front lawn there. I went there multiple times with my dad in Papa Jackson's final years as Dad provided medical care for him. My father's respect and tender affection for his own father as he sat by his bedside holding his frail, slender hand is forever etched in my memory, as is the memory of many good times with the extended family on the front lawn of the "Old Homeplace."

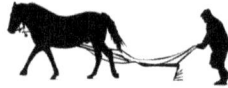

3

GROWING UP AT SAMMY SWAMP

"Come on, fellas! Faster! Faster! We'll never get this corn shelled!" Ralph shouted, trying to push Carl and Robert to feed corn into the sheller more quickly. Flushed and puffing, both he and Scott turned the handle on the corn sheller as fast as they could. Ralph supervised the entire operation as the younger brothers gathered the yellow field corn as fast as their stubby little hands could and tossed it into the wide, open mouth of the sheller. Stripped of every kernel, bare cobs spewed out of the other end — yellow kernels falling into a bucket underneath. Their job wasn't finished until five bushels of corn were shelled. Eventually, the freshly shelled corn was poured into burlap bags, and the tired but exuberant boys lugged the product of their labor to Mr. Brogdon's grist mill, where part of the corn was ground into grits and the rest into meal. Every Saturday, their responsibility turned into an adventure, because the brothers knew they could then spend their weekly twenty-five cents allowance at the store.

All four brothers stared at the assortment of candies and goodies behind the glass counter at Mr. Brogdon's store. Each of them calculated the price of their favorite candy and what could possibly be purchased with their monies. This delightful calculation occurred every Saturday morning as their allowance burned a hole in their pockets. Mr. Brogdon waited and watched patiently as the four Jackson boys carefully deliberated over their weekly purchase. Suddenly, Ralph spoke up, "Can you make change for me, Mr. Brogdon? I need to save a nickel." Both Mr. Brogdon and the three other brothers stared at him in open-mouthed surprise.

"Whatever in the world for, Ralph?" queried the store owner.

"Yeah, why?" the brothers asked in unison.

Hesitantly, Ralph responded, "In a few months we will take up an offering at church for the missionaries overseas. You know — the Lottie Moon Offering at Christmas. I want to start saving a nickel a week until then."

Mr. Brogdon smiled and said, "Well, Ralph, that's a fine thing for you to do."

Ralph smiled broadly like a Cheshire cat. His brothers continued to stare as if suddenly he had grown two heads. Wide-eyed, they looked at each other, rubbed their quarters, glanced longingly at the candy counter, and scuffed their shoes on the floor. Then Scott said a little uncertainly, "I was thinking of doing the same thing. How about y'all?"

Robert and Carl's faces fell. Clutching their quarters tightly, they looked longingly at the candy counter and then at Mr. Brogdon's smiling face. They reluctantly, but unconvincingly, mumbled, "Yeah, we were, too."

Thus began several months of weekly savings, one nickel per week led by big brother Ralph. As their pile of nickels accumulated, so did their excitement about contributing to the Christmas mission offering.

At the Jackson farm, chores started before breakfast. Chores never ended. Work never ended. Everybody in the Jackson family had responsibilities — from the youngest to the oldest, from daybreak to dark. As a subsistence farming family, they worked hard just to make ends meet like many others in Clarendon County. Because of the presence of chickens, cows and pigs, food was always plentiful for the large family — but the livestock required everyday maintenance.

The most difficult time was hog-killing time. Occasionally, their father would kill five hogs in one day. This always had to be done in very cold weather. They killed and butchered the hogs, scraped away the hair, and then hung them by the back legs on a pole. The abdomens were carefully opened, allowing the viscera to pour out into a large tub. The liver was carefully extracted. This would be cooked and mixed with pre-cooked rice and seasoning and then placed into containers to make liver pudding.

The family made their own pork sausage with trimmings from the hogs. Lean meat was mixed with some fat and was ground up by putting it through a sausage mill. When the meat was ground up, seasoned, and thoroughly mixed, it was stuffed into casings. As the sausage meat passed through the grinder, it would then pass through a tube over which the casings had been placed. The meat filled the casings, which were then hung in a smokehouse for about two weeks for the curing process. When cooked, their very own sausage was very tasty. The hog carcasses were left hanging in the smokehouse for two or three days before being taken down and cut into hams, shoulders, and sides. These were packed and covered with salt and left in a large wooden box for about three weeks. Then the pieces of pork were taken out of the salt, rinsed in cold water and hung in the smokehouse, which further cured the meat. When the meat was thoroughly cured, it lasted several months just hanging in the smokehouse. The cured ham was quite tasty.

Robert's older sister Eunice recalls, "We had chicken, eggs, and milk from the cows, but I don't ever recall having any beef when we were growing up. We skimmed the cream off the milk to churn into butter. When the boys brought the bucket of milk to the house, we strained it through a cloth, put it in pans, and let it sit overnight. The cream would rise to the top, we skimmed this off with a spoon. For many years, Mama put the cream into a two-quart jar and shook it until it turned to butter. She removed this from the jar and rinsed it in cold water. She would then put the butter into a small dish, make it into a mound, and go around it with a spoon making little dips. I never could make the butter look like Mama's."

For years, the Jackson family planted sugar cane, which grew into tall stalks, five to six feet tall. When it was mature, the stalks were cut and taken to a syrup mill, where the stalks were crushed and the liquid from them was put into a large vat. The liquid was boiled over a fire for many hours, turning the liquid into cane syrup. After cooking, the syrup was dipped out and put into gallon-sized cans. Biscuits with syrup were standard fare at the Jackson dinner table. The children loved to put a finger into the side of a biscuit and pour syrup into the hole. Papa Jackson especially loved syrup at the end of his meal, putting syrup on his plate and sopping it with his biscuit.

Maintaining a farm also meant plowing, planting, cultivating, harvesting, grinding, and canning. During the summer, the family did a lot of canning of butter beans, peas, tomatoes, corn, and peaches. This was really hard and hot work. Papa Jackson routinely planted sweet potatoes, which were dug up in the fall. He put the potatoes in a small hole that was dug out of the soil — laid pine straw in the hole and then piled the potatoes on top. After a period of time, they were covered with straw and then dirt, creating a potato bank. When sweet potatoes were needed for a meal, a small hole was made in the potato bank and someone had to reach inside and take out the potatoes needed. The hole was then recovered, and the sweet potatoes would last until summertime.

The work never ended, especially in the summertime. One brother, Ralph, recalled:

> Robert, Carl, Scott, and I performed every type of work done on the farm, in addition to shelling the corn. Together we picked up punctured cotton squares, shocked oats and wheat, dropped peas in the cornfields, broke corn into heap rows, turned potato and water-melon vines and picked cotton. We set, poisoned, suckered, topped, hung, cured, took off and laced tobacco. We also hauled in hay and shook the pecan trees. This is just to mention a few of the things we did as boys growing up on the farm. Of course, after the farm chores, we did our homework at night.

Despite the requisite labor, fun-loving boys always made time for some exciting diversions with their boundless energy.

Sally

The early morning dew lay like a blanket on the grass beyond the house while the rooster crowed obnoxiously and continuously. Big Sister Eunice had already stepped out to sweep the hard-packed yard right around the house where no grass grew. Dense, black swarms of gnats hung in midair over the surrounding fields. The early morning heat and humidity combined to make the youngest four Jackson boys break a smooth sweat just walking to the barn. Ralph, the eldest of the four, hitched up Sally the mule to the wagon, while Scott put a galvanized bucket of slop for the pigs on the back of the wagon. Robert, the youngest, and Carl threw out scratch feed for the chickens. Scott, the biggest and the strongest, began to milk the cow. When he finished milking, he carried his pail full of fresh, warm milk to the back porch while Robert and Carl watched from their perch on the back of the wagon.

As soon as Scott touched the back porch and turned to come toward the wagon, Ralph whispered, "Y'all watch this."

"Hee yah, Sally, giddy up."

Startled, ole Sally broke into a trot, jerking the wagon behind her. Robert and Carl smiled and broke into childish laughter. Left behind, Scott frowned and broke into a sprint, not wanting to walk all the way to the pigpen. Sally picked up speed as Ralph flicked the reins and hollered, "Giddy up, Sally!" The wagon lurched down the hard-packed and rutted red clay road. Robert and Carl held on for dear life, still laughing at Scott's struggle to keep up even though he was a fast runner. The wagon fell into a hole, bounced right out, and catapulted the bucket of slop off the rear of the wagon and all over their thoroughly irate brother. Scott never broke stride. He just came on faster and meaner and covered in slop! Nobody laughed now because everybody knew about Scott's temper.

Carl and Robert screamed like little girls. When Ralph saw what had happened, he started flogging Sally, but she was too old and too slow. Seeing big brother Scott about to win this contest, Carl shouted at Robert, "Off! Off! Jump!" And he pushed six-year-old Robert off the wagon. Robert landed on his right leg awkwardly with a loud snap, sort of like a .22-rifle shot. Carl took off through the four-foot-tall corn field like a frightened deer, not to be seen again until lunch time. Ralph kept whipping Sally and hoping for a miracle, while Robert rolled on the ground moaning and holding his right lower leg.

Covered in pig slop, red-faced, breathing hard, and clenching his fists, Scott stood over Robert. Robert whimpered like a whipped pup, holding his leg. Scott looked up as Ralph disappeared; Scott's shoulders slumped and his anger dissipated as he scooped up his baby brother and carried him back to the big house — still covered in pig slop.

The morning frolic ended with a trip to Dr. Harvin and an ACE bandage placed on Robert's ankle for two weeks. The four brothers told that story at family reunions for sixty years, usually starting with, "Hey, Bo, you remember the time the slop bucket jumped off the wagon on top of Scott … ." Every child and grandchild in the family knows that episode by heart.

Barnyard Rodeo

Artesian well water flowed perpetually into a large horse trough in the farm's feed lot. All the livestock watered there. Watching them drink, the four youngest boys fancied themselves to be rodeo riders, riding anything with four legs. How the mules could work all week and let the boys ride them on Saturday and Sunday remains a mystery to the entire family! They liked to ride the hogs, too, and accomplished this by shutting up twenty-five-to-thirty hogs in a large mule pen, running them up into one corner of the pen, then jump-straddling any one they chose. They rode the old sows, the boars, the barrows, and the gilts — none could escape four farm boys looking for a free rodeo ride. Of course, they never told their papa about riding the hogs because this was a big "no-no."

On one occasion, Ralph and Scott said to Robert, "Hey, Bo, let us put you on the old milk cow."

Trusting his older brothers, Robert immediately agreed. Hoisting their younger brother up on the cow, they dropped him onto her back, slapped her on the rear, and shouted, "Yee-haa!" Immediately, she whirled and ran, bucking across the lot. Robert quickly pitched over and face-planted in the soft mud. Thankfully, he wasn't hurt, and they had a big laugh about it; however, no one was foolish enough to try riding the milk cow again.

Shenanigans

Then there was the time Carl caught a garter snake and rolled it up in the cuff of his blue jeans, leaving it there until supper time. Papa Jackson required quiet and decorum at the supper table. Carl sat between Scott and Robert. During supper he dropped his napkin on the floor, leaned over, unrolled his cuff, and dropped that snake in Scott's lap. Scott screamed bloody murder and stood up abruptly, turning the entire dinner table over onto the floor. The floor was covered with food and dishes, while Robert and Carl stared at Papa Jackson, horrified. Papa Jackson never moved an inch. Unruffled, he said to Scott, "Sonny boy, it's just a green snake. Y'all boys clean up this mess."

Mike Epperson tells of the occasion when Scott was sleeping, and Carl and Robert decided to give him the hot foot. They put matches between his toes and lit them with another match. Scott woke up suddenly with red-hot toes, took a big swing, and knocked Robert out cold. When Robert woke up, Scott was cradling his head in his lap, pleading, "Robert, please wake up, wake up."

The Gator Hole and the Boy Scout

At lunchtime most days, while the adults took a nap in the noontime heat, the youngest boys, still full of energy, took off for Sep Harvin's or Morgan Saul's pond for a swim. This particular day broiled as hot as any

Lowcountry, southern day could. The barefoot boys — Scott; Carl; Robert; Mike Epperson, their eldest sister's son who was just a few years younger than Robert, and his friend, Furman Avins — hiked about one mile to Sep Harvin's pond with a warning from their sister Eunice ringing in their ears: "You boys stay out of those gator holes. I don't want to hear of somebody drowning in a gator hole." There weren't really any alligators in any of those ponds, but there were deep holes dangerous to young swimmers and ominously called "gator holes." Constantly fed by an artesian spring even in the hottest, driest summer, the pond was just big enough and deep enough for swimming with a three-foot spillway. Live oaks spread their 100-year-old limbs over the pond, providing shade and a place for rope swings. Perfect for swimming and fishing on hot summer days, the water was always cool, dark, and deep.

The older boys — Scott, Carl, and Robert — swam on one end of the pond, while Mike and Furman hung close to the dam. Robert had just returned from a Boy Scout jamboree in Pennsylvania. He was full of stories about his adventures and all the new things he had learned as a Scout. Even as a twelve-year-old boy, he was an excellent storyteller and captured everyone's attention as he told about the hundreds of young Scouts in attendance and all the seminars he attended. He even wrote an article for *The Manning Times*, his hometown newspaper, detailing the experience.

Suddenly, Furman shouted, "Help, Mike's drowning!" The three uncles looked, and sure enough Mike was under water. He then bobbed up, gasped for breath, and went under again with his arms over his head. Furman shouted, "He's in a gator hole!" Immediately, Robert swam toward Mike lightning fast. Mike bobbed up again, whooped for air, and went down. Three feet away from Mike, Robert dove under the surface, swam under his nine-year-old nephew, grabbed him under the armpits, and propelled him up onto the bank of the pond. Scrambling up beside the weak and lifeless body of his young nephew, Robert began to compress his chest. The others stared at each other in amazement, never having seen anything like that before. In a few moments, Mike gasped, began to cough and then breathed on his own. The color slowly returning to his cheeks, he sat up, smiled weakly and leaned on his uncle Robert. Robert trembled all over from his own exertion and trepidation; his eyes flashed with excitement.

Scott exclaimed, "Robert, wherever in the world did you learn how to do that?"

"At the Boy Scout jamboree," Robert responded through heavy breathing. "It's a new lifesaving technique they taught us. Never thought I'd get to use it so soon."

Carl slapped Robert on the back and said proudly, "Bo, there just ain't no end to you."

Then they all lay back on the green grass in the warm sunshine, ever so proud of their Boy Scout brother. Upon interviewing Mike Epperson at eighty-two years old regarding this event, he stated, "I have no doubt that Uncle Robert saved my life that day." Little did they know as they lay beside the gator hole that another day would come when their baby brother-turned-physician would rescue another one of them from certain death years later.

Coach Howard Comes Recruiting

Then there was the time Coach Frank Howard came from Clemson to recruit Scott to play football. Along with his assistant, he spent the entire afternoon sitting on the front porch talking to Papa Jackson, Eunice, and Scott. Finally, it got close to supper time. Eunice excused herself, went to the kitchen, and said to Robert and Carl, "I declare, I don't believe that coach is going to leave before supper. I'm going to have to feed him and his assistant. Carl, you and Robert catch me a chicken, but do not, under any circumstances, do so in the front yard where Coach Howard can see you catching that yard bird. Do you understand me?" Carl and Robert nodded and set off at a trot.

However, every time they got close to that chicken it had a premonition of what was to come, and it ran right into the front yard. After multiple attempts, that hen made the fatal mistake of running under the front porch where Coach Howard and Papa Jackson sat. The two boys quietly cornered the chicken and brought it proudly to Eunice, who "quick as two shakes of a sheep's tail" had that yard bird fried up and on the table. After supper, Coach Howard said, "Eunice, I do believe that was the best fried chicken I have ever eaten." Of course, she beamed with pleasure and shared his compliment with family and friends for years afterwards.

Scott played four years at Clemson as a tight end, becoming an ACC All Conference player. He also played in the Orange Bowl against Tulane in 1954. When I was a student at Clemson, there was a life-size portrait of my uncle Scott in his uniform running with the football in the old Fike Fieldhouse. I delighted in telling my college friends: "That's my uncle Scott. He was an ACC All Conference tight end and MVP his senior year!" How about that!

When Scott was at Clemson, he experienced shortness of breath and rapid heartbeat that sometimes made him feel dizzy and faint. One Saturday when he was home in Manning, he caught Dr. Harvin, his family doctor, on Main Street and described his symptoms. Dr. Harvin replied, "Scott, I have heard a medical description of these symptoms, but I can't tell you the exact medical term. However, I learned from a heart specialist that if you will squat and hold your breath whenever these symptoms occur, they will shortly go away."

Scott laughed out loud and said, "Oh, pshaw, Dr. Harvin, quit pulling my leg!"

Dr. Harvin responded, "No, I'm serious. Just try that the next time it happens."

The very next week during football practice, Scott experienced the rapid heartbeat and dizziness again. Remembering what Dr. Harvin had recommended, he immediately squatted and held his breath. The other players in the huddle looked at him in dismay. In a few seconds, the rapid heartbeat spontaneously resolved. One of the players asked, "Jackson, are you all right?" His response? "Aw, I'm fine, just following my doctor's orders." Neither he nor his doctor knew it at the time, but he was suffering from SVT — supraventricular tachycardia, which often responds to a Valsalva maneuver, such as squatting and holding one's breath. Not knowing his diagnosis or what therapy was available in the 1950s, Scott had to perform this maneuver multiple times through his college career, and, fortunately, it always worked for him.

At the end of his college career, Scott was invited to participate in the Blue-Gray Game in Knoxville, Tennessee, which was considered a great honor. He and his wife, Roseanne, boarded a train and rode up to Knoxville to participate in that postseason game. All the players were required to undergo a medical evaluation before their participation in the Blue-Gray Game. Scott made the mistake of telling the physician about his rapid heartbeat condition, and the doctor disallowed him from participating. Scott vehemently protested, saying, "But, Doctor, I have had this condition for four years, and it has not hindered my ability to play at all. It always responds to the maneuver recommended by my family doctor. All I have to do is squat and hold my breath." The doctor had never heard of such a thing and would not allow Scott to participate. He and Roseanne were put back on the train and sent back home, much to their chagrin and disappointment. Thirty years later when he related the incident to me, he was still hot about it!

Paratroopers

Robert and Carl squatted in the hayloft of the barn, looking down at the hard-packed red clay fifteen feet below. They both held a bedsheet over their shoulders like paratroopers. By this time, their brother Jimmy was a captain in Europe fighting the Nazis. They had seen news reels at the local theater describing the heroic efforts of the paratroopers who had parachuted into France on D-Day. Enthralled by those descriptions, they now readied themselves to test their own mettle. "You go first," said Carl, looking anxiously at the space between them and the ground.

"No, you go first," Robert responded with equal timidity.

"OK, we'll go together," they agreed. "One, Two Three, JUMP!"

Robert jumped with a loud whoop, while brother Carl wisely stayed behind. Robert's makeshift parachute fluttered uselessly in the air as Robert dropped like a rock. The end result was a broken arm and a cast for six weeks. For thirty years that story was told and retold, with Robert insisting that he was pushed from the hayloft, and Carl just as insistently denying it — with a mischievous smile!

The good, clean fun of those years included playing marbles for hours on the red clay surface of the front yard with finger-drawn lag lines and circles in the dirt. They played baseball endlessly using a tobacco stick for a bat and swinging away at anything that could be thrown — green pears, cans, corn cobs and rolls of twine. Hand-fashioned footballs were thrown about the yard for hours on end. Who knew that these sweaty little boys with dirty bare feet playing ball for hours in the front yard would one day grow up to be prominent citizens in Clarendon County? Carl and Scott became successful farmers right there in Sammy Swamp; Ralph farmed in nearby Gable, South Carolina, and worked for Hartsville Oil Mill (which later became Coker Cottonseed and Oil), while the baby of the family became a much-loved hometown physician.

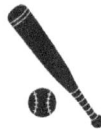

4

AMERICA JOINS THE WAR

While the four youngest Jackson boys (Robert, Carl, Scott, and Ralph) played with marbles, collected chicken eggs, and learned to milk cows, the war in Europe escalated in 1944. Older brothers Jehu and Billy, although otherwise employed, helped operate the farm while their father worked in St. Matthews, South Carolina. They also served in the Home Guard in Manning, whose responsibility was to guard the beaches of South Carolina and the dam on Lake Marion. M.R., the oldest brother, secured a job with the civil service in Panama during the war.

Folks in Clarendon County, like other rural folk around the United States, drove into town on Saturdays to the local theater to watch a movie and newsreels reporting on the war in Europe and the Pacific. In Manning, this happened to be the Hollywood Theater, known to the locals as Ma Green's Theater, located at 35 North Brooks Street and opened by Mr. and Mrs. H.T. Green in 1933. Mr. Green died shortly thereafter, leaving Mrs. Green to operate the theater by herself. "The ticket window opened onto Brooks Street. A pot-bellied stove, providing heat for the entire building, sat to the right as patrons entered the theater. The projection room was on the second story where, when he became old enough, their son, Tommy Green, ran the projector and changed reels. On at least one occasion, the fast-moving film caught fire, causing an intermission as the fire was extinguished and a new reel threaded."

News reports of the swift advance of the Third Armored Division of the

United States First Army, also known as the Spearhead Division, electrified the nation. The division landed in Normandy after D-Day in late June of 1944 and "spearheaded" its way through northern France, all the way to the German border by mid-September — liberating dozens of cities in France and capturing 76,720 German soldiers, but also sustaining 9,243 battle casualties and 2,147 deaths (this number varies a little per source). The division claimed to be the first to fire an "American field artillery shell onto German soil of the war." During the Battle of Saint-Lo — a notable battle — the division faced the dilemma of heavy fighting among hedgerows, or earthen embankments. "Crossing the hedgerows necessitated exposing the vulnerable underbellies of the tanks, making them susceptible to enemy fire. The engineers and maintenance crews ingeniously took the large I-beams from the invasion barriers used on the beaches at Normandy and welded them onto the front of the Sherman tanks as crossing rams. The tanks were then able to strike the hedgerows at high speed, breaking through them without exposing their vulnerable underbellies. Without this innovation, the tanks could not get through or across the hedgerows." After refitting and resting in Belgium, they eventually assisted in the capture of Cologne on March 7, 1945, after reaching the Rhine River. On April 11, 1945, they found the Dora-Mittelbau concentration camp and liberated the prisoners, transporting 250 to a hospital.

In the middle of this rapid advance and activity was Lieutenant Jimmy Jackson, the fourth oldest Jackson brother. Lieutenant Jackson — an ROTC graduate from Clemson College turned Army officer, and later promoted to captain — commanded over fifty men, many of whom were much older than his twenty years of age. He commented in a letter home to his father: "The responsibility of leading fifty men is heavy. Some of them are as old as thirty-eight, but they never question my commands." Jimmy was wounded twice — once in the back and arm, and later in the thigh in a subsequent incident. Both wounds were shrapnel wounds, and both required extended stays in the hospital for surgery and recuperation. Never removed, the shrapnel remained in his thigh as a souvenir of the war for the rest of his life. He received the Purple Heart with two oak-leaf clusters for his battlefield injuries. He was also awarded the Bronze Star for bravery on the battlefield.

His father's spiritual influence over Jimmy's life was obvious in many of his letters home, which often closed with a request for prayer for "my safe return home if it's the Lord's will." On January 10, 1945, he wrote his father from Belgium, requesting, "You must ask all of the family to pray for me that I may come through safely, if it is the Lord's will, and I will always remember the verse that you like so well: 'The Lord is my shepherd, I shall not want … .' "

In every letter home, he inquired about his father's health and about the crops. He asked about his brothers and Eunice and Edna, particularly the younger brothers, whom he referred to as "the boys." He closed with, "Don't you worry about me. I'll be fine."

He wrote his sister Eunice on March 4, 1945, after returning to Germany trying to catch up to his division, which had just reached the Rhine River at Cologne: "I'm looking forward to getting back to the fellows that I have fought with now twice before … . Now, Eunice, please don't worry about me because I'm going to be fine. All we can do is to trust in God and pray, and that if it's His will I shall be returned just as I left. I have my complete trust and faith in Him because I know Him as my personal Savior and Friend."

In a letter home to his dad in 1944, presaging his future educational expertise, Jimmy wrote regarding his expectations of the four youngest brothers' scholastic achievements: "How's Robert, Scott, Carl, and Ralph doing in school? I suppose Robert is still making high marks. You should try to get him to study hard so that he will be at the head of his class. I believe that he can do it. Scott and Carl, though, they will just get by."

On May 17, 1944, *The Manning Times* included the following letter Uncle Jimmy wrote while he was at Camp Robertson, Arkansas, in memory of his mother, who passed away in 1937:

This letter is dedicated with deepest devotion to my mother, to your mother, wherever she may be, and to all mothers who have sons in the service. — Lieutenant W.S. "Jimmy" Jackson

Mother Dear: You always were a little embarrassed on Mother's Day. I remember … "Such a fuss!" you used to say, hiding your face for a moment in the roses we children sent to you. But you always wore one of the roses to church, and as you sat beside Father on the hard, brown bench, your face was warm with a secret brightness. You never threw the roses away until the petals fell in a scarlet shower on the piano top. And you kept all the silly cards we sent you.

This year, though, no card can say all I want to say. So, you'll find this note tucked in the box among the roses.

There is no card that explains how all the sights and sounds and feelings of our lives are woven into our memory of you. The smell of the lilac bush at the corner of the steps and the fragrance of cookies … that, somehow, Mother, is you. The slam of the screen door, hurrying footsteps, laughter, and sometimes silence … that is you. The crease in the tablecloth, snow-white curtains, the shaded quiet of a sick room … that is you, Mother.

Mother, you know a child remembers a great many things more than grown-ups, I suppose. There was the dirt road in front of our house, long and steep for wagon rides … and always, at the end of the road, when the last ride was over, you were waiting. It was good to walk, puffing and tired, up the path at dusk, and see you at the lighted window, head bent over the sewing box.

Do you remember the lamp you brought home, the one with the heavy silver base? We used to make faces into its polished surfaces, and gasp with laughter at the reflections sent back to us. When you would scold us after that, it helped to remember that you could make the funniest faces of all.

The first day we marched off to school, leather satchels slung proudly over our shoulders … remember? I still can feel the warmth of your breath on the back of my neck as you leaned over to fix my shirt. I can still see you on the porch, waiting for us to come back. I still remember, Mother, the frowns you gave as we trailed mud across the kitchen floor … the smudge of flour in the edge of your hair … the way your hands lay tiredly on your lap sometimes. None of these have been forgotten.

Lodged in the crevices of our minds are some words you said when we were old enough to listen. "What's the use of this," I used to ask as I struggled over my lessons. "Nothing you do is lost," you scolded lightly. "You'll never get anywhere unless you finish what you start."

And once, I remember you said, "Whatever else you may do or say, you must have 'faith in faith,' or you will have no anchor to hold to in this world." Your wisdom, Mother, has become our wisdom, in a way, and your faith our faith.

Sadly, Robert never knew his and Jimmy's mother, but his brother's exemplary military service was, no doubt, an influence on Robert's patriotic fervor and a harbinger of things to come.

5

A RISING STAR

As intense and as serious as ever, Robert stared earnestly into Abbot's brown eyes. They sat on a blanket at the end of a long corn row at the bottom of a hill — invisible from the Jackson farmhouse. A mule with a plow attached stood patiently nearby, swishing flies with his tail. Robert plowed down and back over the hill, stopped and drank sweet tea with Abbot, then resumed his plowing. He wasn't the only Jackson boy who had discovered this trick. Scott and Roseanne and Carl and Margaret had met at this same spot on many occasions to drink a little sweet tea and discuss future plans.

Robert and Abbot first met at a Manning High School basketball game in November 1951. Abbot had just entered the eighth grade. Robert was only a tenth grader but had already begun to show exceptional leadership ability recognized by both teachers and classmates alike. They began an on-and-off three-year courtship that was rather stormy, with frequent episodes of "breaking up." However, they always "made up" eventually and continued to make plans for their future together. Robert never spoke of any occupation other than becoming a physician.

At the end of the corn row while holding Abbot's hand tightly, Robert declared, "I just know in my heart that God intends for me to be a medical doctor. I don't know how I am going to accomplish it, but I plan to go to Clemson, then to medical school in Charleston. After school, I'll come right back here to Manning and open a medical practice. Maybe I could work with Dr. Harvin. Wouldn't that be something! Why don't you come with me?"

That was big talk for a poor farm boy, the son of a dirt farmer, the youngest of ten children. College scholarships were rare in those days. The children of the wealthy went to professional schools. Robert had the academic ability but no financial capability.

Abbot stared dreamily into his intense, hazel eyes, believing every word, never doubting that Robert could accomplish anything he set his mind to, and willing to sacrifice her educational and personal goals to help him accomplish his. Then, as now, the surest path to poverty was to leave school early and marry without an education, which was exactly what she was contemplating. Nevertheless, she was confident that she was hitching her wagon to a rising star.

Robert excelled at everything he put his hands to. He became the vice president and then the president of his class at Manning High School. He was an officer in every organization he joined and excelled in every sport. Indeed, the staff of the *Monarch*, the Manning High School annual, honored him with the following:

Robert Jackson has been selected by the *Monarch* staff as Boy of the Year (1953-1954).

Robert was chosen because of his outstanding curricular activities in Manning High during his senior year. Robert has served as president of the student body and student council for the '53-'54 school term. King Teen, Sports Editor of the *Mahiscan*, member of the Block M Club, and a senior superlative are some of the other honors and offices Robert has held this year.

In the athletic department, Robert must again be recognized as a leader and good sport. He was basketball co-captain, right tackle of the football team, and catcher of the baseball team.

After winning the oratorical contest at Manning High and the district contest, he competed in the K. of P. [Knights of Pythias] contest and won third place. The *Monarch* salutes Robert for his outstanding work this year and congratulates him on all of his achievements.

As mentioned, in the sports arena, Robert played tackle on the football team at 145 pounds (an adequate weight in the 1950s). Downright aggressive at that position, he was offered a partial football scholarship to Wofford College — which he declined because his goal was medicine, not football. Under his picture in the high school annual where he wore his football uniform, the caption reads "Field General." I inquired about this on one occasion as I flipped through the annual and laughed at pictures of my parents as children often do. "Dad, what's a field general?"

"A field general is the guy who calls the plays."

I persisted with, "I thought you were a tackle, not a quarterback."

He responded, "That's right."

I questioned him further. "How come you called the plays?"

With a twinkle in his eye, he replied, "The quarterback couldn't remember all of the plays, and I could — so the coach designated me the play caller. Hence, the title 'field general.'"

As was often the case with my dad, I didn't know if he was telling me the truth or pulling my leg until my mom confirmed it. Whoever heard of such!

As I laughed my way through his high school annual, my dad relayed the following story regarding his basketball exploits. "We were playing in a conference title game. I was positioned as a guard — why, I don't know, because I could never dribble very well. I noticed the opposing team brought the ball up the floor, passing it back and forth between two guards with the same rhythm every time. I thought to myself, *I can bide my time and easily surprise them with a steal and then an easy layup.* In the second half, we were down by four points and time was running out. I decided it was time to go for it. As the opposing team brought the ball up the floor with the same passing rhythm, I ran forward at the half-court line, surprised them easily, stole the ball, dribbled twice, and made an easy layup. This was not normal for me, so the home team fans went crazy. On their very next possession, I executed the same maneuver for two more points. Our fans were jubilant. The opposing team was rattled, and the game was now tied. Two possessions later, the game was still tied. Their guards lapsed into that same rhythm as they brought the ball up the court. I made a break for it, snatched the ball out of the air, dribbled twice on a dead run, and made another easy layup. My heart pounded and the fans screamed. The clock ran out and we won by two points."

"Wow, Dad, that's amazing!"

Then he assumed a pseudo-serious tone, looked me dead in the eye, and said, "Son, that was the only bright spot in my entire basketball career. I was really a pretty sorry basketball player." Then he laughed, and we resumed our perusal of his high school annual.

Considering baseball his best sport in school, Robert played catcher for the Manning High School baseball team, and he also played American Legion baseball for Post 15 in Sumter, South Carolina, along with a number of other athletes from Clarendon County. In 1952, Post 15 won the state championship. One of his teammates was Bobby Richardson, who played shortstop (and probably other positions) for the team. Bobby Richardson hailed from Sumter, South Carolina, and signed on with the Yankees the day he graduated from high school on June 12, 1953. He still holds several records and is arguably the "greatest all-time Yankee second baseman after Hall of Famer Tony Lazzeri."

I was able to speak with Bobby Richardson and John Duffie, both of whom played on that state championship-winning Post 15 team. Both in their early eighties, they are in good health at this writing and have excellent recollections of that season. The team beat Greenwood four out of seven games to win the championship. According to Mr. Duffie, they then participated in a four-team regional tournament in Florence, South

Carolina. They lost the first game, and everyone thought they were out of the tournament. However, they won the rest of the games to triumph in the regional contest. Post 15 then competed in the sectional tournament in Charleston, South Carolina, against teams from Memphis, Tennessee, and Austin, Texas. Unfortunately, they did not prevail at that level. When they returned home, the mayor of Sumter arranged a parade for the team. They all rode into town on a bright red fire truck, and received a golden baseball on a chain and keys to the city.

Both John and Bobby remembered Robert and Abbot immediately. Invariably, folks have fond memories of Robert Jackson, and such was the case with his former Post 15 teammates. When I relayed my identity on the phone, Bobby Richardson immediately responded, "I know exactly who you are. I remember your father and Abbot quite well. He was a wonderful teammate, and I enjoyed competing with him."

John Duffie recalled immediately, "Yes. Yes. I recall Robert and Abbot. I was a Clemson cheerleader in the days when they only had male cheerleaders. I didn't have a car, so Robert and Abbot took me to Georgia to cheer and see his brother Scott play football on one of the hottest days ever. He drove us there in his '39 Ford. Robert was the nicest, most polite fellow student. He was lively and full of energy. Abbot was great with child. Don't know how she stood the heat.

"Everyone thought well of Robert. When he first joined our baseball team, he was so proud of his brother Scott, who played football for Clemson. He would walk up to any newcomer and ask, 'Do you know my brother, Scott Jackson? You know he plays football for Clemson!'

"Your dad was so much fun to be around. I remember he was a very aggressive player, although not very big in size. Coach Hutch would point him out and say, 'It's not the size of the dog in the fight, but the size of the fight in the dog.' I still remember Coach saying that to this day.

"Your dad was not the only player from Clarendon County on the Post 15 team that year. Bill Arant was from Manning. He was co-captain of the team and played first base. Jack Hodge was from Alcolu and played left field. Pete Gibson was our starting pitcher, and he was from Summerton. Our other pitchers, Richard Bradham and Bobby Richardson, were both from Sumter. Of course, Bobby was best known for playing second base or shortstop. Don Frierson was from Olanta and played third base. You realize our Post 15 state championship was really a Sumter and Clarendon County team."

Seventeen years later, that Post 15 team held a reunion (Mickey Mantle Day at Riley Park, June 28, 1969) in Sumter, South Carolina, as part of a fundraiser for the ballpark. The 1952 state championship team, which included Dad, played the 1969 Post 15 team, and beat them in seven innings. I saw it with my own eyes. Bobby Richardson had also arranged for Mickey Mantle and Tony Kubek — who played with him on the New York Yankee World Series championship teams of 1958, 1961, and 1962 — to be present and to participate in a home-run hitting contest. I remember the event vividly for two reasons. First, just watching the great Mantle hit "blue darters" into left field thrilled my soul. (According to *The Sumter Daily Item*, Mantle had refused to hit any balls since his retirement the previous fall, but for some reason he chose to do so on this occasion for the begging and screaming crowd.) Second, and more pertinent to my growing interest in medical science, I saw my first case of neurofibromatosis, also known as Von Recklinghausen's disease, as we sat in the stands marveling at Mickey and Tony. I noticed a woman with bulbous tumors on her bare arms, neck, and face. As a teenager, I couldn't stop staring. Finally, I whispered to my doctor dad, "Dad, what's wrong with that woman on my right?"

He barely cut his eyes to the right, resumed watching the home-run hitting contest, and responded casually, "She has von Recklinghausen's disease."

Well, I was incredulous, and a little indignant, that he would presume to make a diagnosis — especially with a highfalutin name like that with just a casual glance. I retorted immediately, "How do you know that? You didn't even hardly look at her."

His response was classic, a response I have used with my own children innumerable times, much to their dismay: "Trust me, Son. There are just some things I know."

On June 4, 1954, Manning High School held a graduation ceremony with the theme of "Youth's Hope for Tomorrow." As president of the student body, Robert made a speech entitled "Peace with Freedom." He received multiple awards — including the leadership award, the most outstanding athlete award, and a declamation medal for participating successfully in a declamation contest in which he won regional honors.

◆　◆　◆　◆　◆

While seated on that blanket sipping iced tea in the shade at the end of a long corn row, Robert finished dazzling Abbot with his plans for college and medical school. She was fully prepared to follow him anywhere, even if that meant foregoing her own college dreams and working hard to put him through school. Their plans were sealed, so after his graduation, they drove to Kingstree, South Carolina, twenty miles away, to be married. Their plan was to keep it a secret until the end of summer and then make an announcement that they had been married all summer and were going to college together. Alas, the best laid plans of mice and men often go awry. Driving back into Manning, Abbot's mom, Anne Land, spotted them driving into town formally dressed at eleven o'clock on a Monday morning, when Robert should have been on the farm driving a tractor and Abbot should have been at her job at the telegraph office. Suddenly, the cat was out of the bag, and the truth had to be told. Robert had no money, so he planned to drop Abbot off at her home, which was accomplished after a long explanation to Abbot's parents. His brothers felt sorry for him and took up an offering of forty dollars so he and Abbot could go on a short honeymoon to Pawleys Island. My mom relayed to me many years later that one morning on their honeymoon, my dad saw his reflection in the semi-darkness in a full-length mirror on the back of the bathroom door. Supposing there was an intruder, he threw a punch, breaking the mirror and injuring his hand. Of course, he had to protect his new bride.

Abbot's parents, Anne and Calhoun (Coon) Land loved Robert and supported them all the way. They were worried about how they would make it financially, but the young couple worked and made money that summer of 1954, setting aside enough money to last until Christmas. With great expectations and a certain amount of anxiety, they set off for Clemson in September in a black 1939 Ford coupe, which Robert's brother Ralph had restored and Abbot's parents had bought for them.

John Duffie concluded with the statement, "Your mother is quite a remarkable woman. The way she worked to put your dad through college and medical school, while at the same time having several babies, was amazing. Nobody thought they would make it, but they did — and it is to your mother's credit that she supported your father so well. A lesser woman would have thrown in the towel along the way. I know you must be as proud of your mother as you are of your dad."

By this time, I was smiling all over. I had experienced that same conversation with a dozen other folks already in the writing of this book — both family and friends. Everyone recognized Abbot's extraordinary contribution to Robert's professional goals and to holding the family together while he was in medical training, during the arduous early years of medical practice, and while he was away in Southeast Asia. *You may ask where she came by such fortitude?*

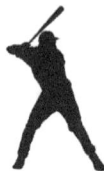

6

ABBOT

Rolling like logs and laughing like the adolescents we were, my sister Anne and I threw ourselves under the pews from the back of the sanctuary all the way down the incline to the front. Over and over we spun and twisted for what seemed like hours while Mom perfected the Sunday morning anthem and the First Baptist Church of Manning resounded with the majestic strains of the great hymns of the Christian faith. I've often wondered if God was laughing and enjoying the moment as much as we did. The memory is certainly precious to me, not so much the rolling, but the recollection of Mama practicing the organ and then playing on Sunday mornings. Even better was when she practiced the piano in our living room at home. That is how I got my start as a singer, standing behind Mama at the piano and singing gospel songs provided by Mr. Simmons, the music director at our church and my first voice instructor.

After helping Dad through college and medical school and then rearing her children, Mom continued her own education. She first obtained her GED, then began taking college classes in January 1969 after my youngest brother Richard started elementary school. In fact, I came home from school one day and found her at her desk in the den leaning over a pile of books.

"What you doing, Mom?"

"I'm studying."

Surprised, I asked, "Studying what?"

She responded promptly, "English literature."

"How come?"

"I'm going to college!"

And that was that!

After more than fourteen years of marriage and at the age of thirty, still looking like a college girl, Mama was a college co-ed. Often, I heard my dad exclaiming proudly about his college girl wife and her excellent grades. Eventually, in 1975 she graduated from Francis Marion College in Florence, South Carolina, with a B.A. degree in English Literature with collaterals in psychology and sociology. She was good at psycho-analyzing her children — called "psycholyzing" by our dad. She began teaching English at Manning Christian Academy, much to the chagrin of my two younger brothers who never managed to become the teacher's pets. They assured me that our mother was the most demanding and strictest teacher they ever encountered. Many times I overheard them grousing about Mom's English class and her high expectations while secluded in their bedroom.

My mom inherited from her progenitors the necessary traits for overcoming adversity and achieving success. I love to tell people that Pocahontas is my grandmother, so here's the story:

On April 5, 1614, a pious English farmer living in Jamestown, Virginia, received permission from the governor to marry an intrepid young Indian woman who had been held in captivity by English settlers for nearly a year. In his letter to the governor, he expressed his love for her and his belief that he would be saving her soul through the institution of Christian marriage. The English farmer was none other than John Rolfe, and the young captive was Matoaka, better known as Pocahontas. Tricking Pocahontas into boarding one of Argall's ships, Captain Samuel Argall's indigenous allies captured her during the first Anglo-Powhatan War. She was then held for ransom, demanding release of English prisoners and supplies held by Powhatan. During her year of captivity, a minister named Alexander Whitaker instructed her in Christianity and taught her English through reading the Bible. Eventually, she was baptized as a Christian and given the name Rebecca.

In March of 1614, before she married Rolfe, violence broke out between hundreds of English settlers and Powhatan's men. Pocahontas was allowed to speak to her father, who was a tribal leader of Algonquin-speaking tribes. She served as mediator between the English and her father. To Powhatan's surprise, she made it clear she preferred to stay with the English settlers. Who knows what kind of dismay that caused around the campfire?

Ultimately, she married John Rolfe and gave birth to Thomas Rolfe on January 30, 1615. Their marriage created a time of peace between the settlers and Powhatan's men.

One of the stated objectives of the Virginia Company was to bring the gospel message to the American Indians. Rebecca Rolfe became a symbol of Indian religious conversion. For this reason, the company decided to bring her to England as a symbol of the transformative power of the gospel and the successful accomplishment of their charter. Presented as an Indian princess, "Matoaka, alias Rebecca, daughter of the most powerful prince of the Powhatan empire of Virginia," she was treated respectfully and even introduced to the king of England at Whitehall Palace.

Rebecca Rolfe contracted a grave illness upon the return voyage to Virginia and died en route in 1617. Before departing from the coastal waters, they went ashore at Gravesend, England, where she was buried at St. George's Church. Members of a number of prominent Virginia families trace their roots back to Pocahontas and John Rolfe through their son, Thomas. Indeed, Dr. Jackson's future wife, Abbot, can call Matoaka, this same Pocahontas, as her ninth great-grandmother. Some say Pocahontas saved the life of John Smith when he was about to be executed by her father, but the story is questioned by some historians.

Then there was Edith Bolling, another woman in Abbot's lineage, known for her strength of resolve and courage. One of the first females to obtain a driver's license and to drive an electric car in Washington, DC, she married Norman Galt in 1896. He died in 1908, leaving Edith his jewelry business, for which she eventually hired a manager while she traveled to Europe — an unusually brave undertaking for a woman of that day, but then she was a rather intrepid young lady.

Seven years later, Edith was introduced to President Woodrow Wilson, who had recently lost his wife. President Wilson fell madly in love with Edith. She agreed to marry after a proper year of mourning had passed. Interestingly, the *Washington Post* of December 19, 1915, headlined "Bride's Ancestry United Old English Aristocracy with Indian Princess." Another newspaper headline read, "White House Bride's Ancestry Traced Back Six Centuries, Includes Indian Princess and Leaders in the War of Roses." Of course, this Indian princess was Pocahontas.

After their marriage, contrary to her confessed disinterest in politics, Edith became her husband's main confidant and "sounding board." After World War I, while on a cross country train to campaign for ratification of the League of Nations, President Wilson suffered a stroke, leaving his mind intact but paralyzing him on one side. In *My Memoir*, Edith's autobiography, she wrote that his advisors cautioned against his resignation at that precarious time and encouraged Edith to be a steward of his health and serve as the go-between for Senators, department secretaries and the president. "She read, digested, and condensed all correspondence before presenting it to him for approval or rejection. No one saw the president without her permission, and she was always present to ensure he did not become overly excited or exhausted." These actions have caused many historians to refer to Edith as "the first female president of the United States" and to call this period "The Petticoat Presidency." She lived for forty-three years after Wilson's death, dying at the age of eighty-nine.

In Abbot's ancestry, civic and government service was primary in the Rolfe, Bolling, and Randolph families. Strong, capable, and intelligent women worked behind the scenes in many of these families — just like Abbot.

♦ ♦ ♦ ♦ ♦

Abbot's mother, Anna Abbot Weisiger, was no less courageous. Raised in Powhatan, Virginia, she graduated from Harrisonburg State Teacher's College (now James Madison University) with a certificate to teach science, English, history, and home economics. Anna obtained a job teaching home economics at the high school in Manning, South Carolina, two states away from her home. Without hesitation, she boarded a train and set off for South Carolina to become a schoolteacher. Arriving at the train depot in Manning, she walked several blocks with her suitcase in hand and moved into the Rigby boarding home on Brooks Street.

Anna walked to school every day through the middle of downtown Manning, requiring her to go right past the Sinclair service station operated by Calhoun "Coon" Land. He immediately noticed the tall, raven-haired beauty and finagled a date utilizing the services of his best friend Bubba Levi, since he was too shy to do so himself. Anna moved back to Virginia after that academic year, whereupon they began two years of correspondence. At some point in time, Anna became "Anne." Coon and Anne married during the Great Depression in 1933 in Virginia; sadly, no one from Manning could afford to attend the wedding except for Bubba Levi. They returned to Manning and ultimately bought a home on Church Street in 1938, where they raised their two children, Anna Abbot Land and John Calhoun Land III.

Some of my fondest memories include hanging out with Granddaddy Land at his Sinclair gas station in downtown Manning. He operated it along with his brother, my uncle Charles Land. He employed a man by the name of Wallace Brunson, a mechanic and a well-known personality himself in the business district of Manning. Granddaddy often gave me a nickel to obtain an ice-cold Orange Crush from the old drink machine that held the drinks suspended by the neck of the bottle. With great delight, I would slide my Orange Crush along the slot out of the machine, then pop the cap off using the bottle opener on the side of the machine. I sat on a wooden

Coca-Cola crate beside Granddaddy and Uncle Charles as we watched the traffic go by on Main Street. In the summertime, I was always barefoot and occasionally made the mistake of stepping on someone's discarded but still burning cigarette butt, burning the fire out of my bare foot. I still remember Granddaddy and Uncle Charles laughing until tears ran down their cheeks while I danced around like a wild Comanche Indian.

I asked my mom how much gas cost when she and Dad started his medical practice, to which she responded, "I don't even know, because all I ever did was pull up to my father's gas station and say, 'Fill 'er up,' and Wallace would fill up my tank. That was your grandfather's contribution to our early married life, to Robert's education, and, later, to his burgeoning medical practice. The only time I had to pay for gas was when we lived in Clemson."

◆　◆　◆　◆　◆

A certain man in Abbot's ancestry demands our attention, Captain Ceth Smith Land, Abbot's great-grandfather, conspicuous for gallantry in the bloody Civil War conflict known as the Battle of the Crater. Twice wounded during the conflict, Captain Land was promoted to major of the regiment for his valor. Judge J.H. Hudson of Bennettsville, South Carolina, lieutenant colonel of the Twenty-Sixth South Carolina regiment, wrote of Major Land, "He was possessed of great powers of endurance, was never sick, always ready for duty, and was cheerful, contented and happy, a jolly companion, a gay soldier, a good fighter, a good disciplinarian but kind to his men and zealous of their rights."

Ceth returned home after the war and immediately applied himself to repairing his ruined fortunes with industry and wise management. He succeeded beyond his expectations. Before the war in September of 1860, he married Miss Mary Jane Thigpen with whom he fathered three children — John Calhoun (who was Coon's father and Abbot's grandfather), Ceth Smith Jr., and Dora Ada.

Major Land acquired many acres of land about ten miles from Manning, South Carolina. This was such beautifully wooded country that he named the place Foreston and built a little town there with streets, stores, etc. Because he had established his home there, he declined to sell the land, building other homes and renting them to a select group of people — people he considered good for the community. His farming operations were extensive; he was very successful in the mercantile business and went far in the turpentine business. He owned and operated the first railroad in Clarendon County, which ran from Lanes to Foreston. People from Sumter and all the surrounding towns had to go to Foreston to get their freight shipments. There was a small town near Foreston that had never been named. The people of this little town prevailed upon Major Land to let his train stop there, but he refused because the town had no name; however, he stated that he would do this if they would name the town. At about that time, Horace Greeley passed through this little town, so they named it in his honor — Greeleyville. From then on, they received their freight shipments at Greeleyville. During his lifetime, Major Land gave each of his children a home completely furnished, a farm, and a business lot in Foreston when they married.

With intrepid and industrious forebears such as these described above, is it any wonder that Abbot was held in such high esteem by all who watched in admiration as she held her little family together during very difficult years? Our mom is just as much a hero to me and my siblings as is our dad. As I often tell her, "You're the best mom we've ever had!" She replies, "I'm the *only* mom you've ever had." I just smile and say, "Yea, that, too, and we wouldn't trade you for any other."

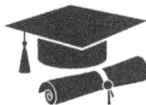

7

COLLEGE AND MED SCHOOL

Robert and Abbot set off for Clemson College in a 1939 Ford sedan with enough money for six months of school and living expenses. They had worked hard the summer of 1954, setting aside several hundred dollars that hopefully would carry them through until summer.

According to Abbot, "Robert and I had heard so many times by now, 'You'll never make it,' that we determined we would make it and in record time. Subsequently, Robert applied to and was accepted into medical school after only three years at Clemson. He did not receive his Clemson college degree until after he graduated from medical school. In later years, it was amusing to observe patients puzzling over his diplomas in his medical office since the graduation date on his medical school diploma is three days earlier than on his college diploma:

Doctor of Medicine
Medical College of South Carolina
June 1, 1961

And then:

Bachelor of Science in Pre-Medicine
Clemson College
June 4, 1961

"Why we weren't scared out of our wits by this tremendous under-taking, I don't quite understand to this day. We only knew that God wanted Robert to be a doctor, and somehow we would achieve that goal."

The birth of their first two children while at Clemson cast serious doubt on their ability to attend medical school. However, their dear friend and family doctor, William H. Hunter, was a constant source of encouragement. Abbot went to his office to determine if a second baby was on the way. "He confirmed my suspicions, which released a flood of tears and created a despair that we could not attend medical school now that we would have two children. I'll never forget the lecture I received that day. Seeing my despair, Dr. Hunter immediately responded, 'Yes, you will go to medical school! If you do, I won't charge you one cent for delivering this baby — but if you don't, this delivery will cost you $300." (In 1956, $300 would be like $3,000 to us today.)

After the first year of college, Robert drove a kerosene truck for Abbot's uncle Oliver Land to make money for the next year of college. Abbot sold ads for a state fair booklet, and she also worked as a waitress for the Accent Restaurant located on Highway 301 next to the Paddock Motel. Back at Clemson, Robert and Abbot held various part-time jobs to make ends meet — Robert, at an insurance company inviting students to come down out of the dorms to meet with an insurance agent and as a waiter at the Clemson House Hotel; and Abbot, as a product demonstrator at a local grocery store on Saturday mornings.

Due to Robert's diligence and academic achievement, he left for medical school after only three years at Clemson. He and Abbot moved to Charleston, South Carolina, in June 1957 to begin medical school with a two-year-old son, Robert E. Jackson Jr. ("Robin," so folks wouldn't call me "Little Robert" — although it didn't stop people from calling me "Little Doc" later in life), and a four-month-old daughter named Anne Land, also called "Sugar" because I couldn't properly say my "little baby sister." I could only say, "My little baby Sugar." The name stuck, much to Anne's chagrin when she became a teenager. Even now, our adult cousins will ask how Sugar and the boys are doing, making us laugh out loud every time — especially since, with a Lowcountry drawl, it is usually pronounced "Shugah."

The summer before medical school, Abbot worked at a local bank in Charleston, and Robert obtained a hot, outside job on a road-paving crew. With both of them working, they could afford childcare for the children. They found an apartment in Robert Mills Manor — a fancy title for the city's low-income housing project where residents paid rent according to their income. Robert and Abbot's monthly rent was seventeen dollars. Years later, Abbot laughingly said, "Our income was so meager, they should have paid us to live there." Many other medical student families lived in the "project," so they soon had a close-knit group of friends riding in the same leaky financial boat.

At some point during Robert's first year of medical school, his brother Scott introduced him to Isabel Weinberg, who lived near Panola out on Highway 261 near his hometown. Mrs. Weinberg had taken an interest in Robert's desire to go to medical school and pledged to send him financial support on a monthly basis. Robert promised that, when his finances improved, he would pay her back. Her response to him: "Robert Jackson, I will accept no reimbursement. I just want you to do the same for some other student one day," which is exactly what he did for multiple other students as time passed. The phrase we use today is "paying it forward." Abbot's brother, my uncle John Land, told me that my dad helped him to purchase a red Volkswagen beetle and helped pay his tuition to college and eventually law school. John Land was not the first or only student for whom Dad paid college tuition. Many years later after her husband was deceased, Mrs. Weinberg's home in Panola caught fire and burned to the ground. Notified that her home was on fire, Dad quickly drove to the scene, where he comforted his benefactor as they watched the flames consume her beloved, longtime residence — which included the many valuable artifacts she had accumulated during her world travels. After she composed herself, Dad gingerly tucked her in his car and drove her back to town to the home of her sister. She later invested in My Lady's Shoppe, a ladies' apparel business in Manning that became quite popular.

After Robert began medical school in September, Abbot took a job as operating room secretary at the medical college hospital, making it possible for them to drive to work and school together, even meeting for lunch on occasion. Robert jokingly told his friends that Abbot gave him twenty-five cents a day for his lunch, and he always brought her change. That may have been a slight exaggeration, but the fact was they lived on an amazingly low income — Abbot's salary of $175 a month and whatever Robert could scrape up selling blood at $25 as often as he was allowed to give. It was not unusual for them to run out of money a week before Abbot's next paycheck was due and before Robert could give blood again. On one occasion, their housekeeper told Abbot, "Ms. Jackson, we have no more sugar or milk." Abbot told her they would have to make do for another week until her paycheck was due. The next morning, the kind-hearted and generous housekeeper stepped off the bus with a bag of groceries she had bought to tide them over until payday.

Robert soon established himself as the wit of his medical school class, joking about everything, including his cadaver "Sarah." As he progressed through anatomy class, the smell of formaldehyde was forever permeating his books, his clothing, and, Abbot thought, even his skin.

The intensity with which Robert studied always amazed Abbot. He made a little study room in a small closet beneath the stairs of their apartment and spent untold hours bent over his plyboard desk in a straight-back chair with a gooseneck lamp shining on his notes and books. He would seldom agree to attend the dances and parties held for the students. When they did go, he would always take his "big Pepsi," so he and Abbot would have a non-alcoholic beverage to drink. He endured much teasing over the fact that he would not take even one drink of alcohol. His often-stated motto was, "If you don't drink the first drop, you won't get drunk." The influence of his father, his sister Eunice, and his Baptist upbringing never left him.

In his freshman physiology class, Robert remembered an event from his days at Clemson that caused some consternation for one of his physiology professors. The story goes like this:

A beloved zoology instructor at Clemson named Professor Ware, whom the students affectionately called Frog Ware, told his zoology class that a local farmer named Mr. Turner had called him, stating that his daughter had swallowed something while swimming in a river near his home. He told Frog Ware emphatically that this "something" kept swimming up into the back of her throat. Laughing, Professor Ware told him, "Next time it swims up, grab it and call me," not taking his story very seriously. Shortly thereafter, Mr. Turner called him back, saying, "Professor Ware, I've got it. Would you please come and take a look?" Professor Ware promptly went to his home and pulled a water snake out of this little girl's gullet.

When Robert told this story to his class, the professor rebuked him for telling tall tales in class. Indignant, Robert stalked out of the classroom, got into his '39 Ford, and drove five hours to Clemson. From the bulletin board outside of Frog Ware's office, he retrieved a newspaper article telling the story of Frog Ware, the little girl the article dubbed "Thankful Turner," and the water snake pulled from her throat. Robert turned around, drove five hours back to Charleston in the same day, and delivered that newspaper article to his professor in front of the entire class the next morning. Indignant, he told his professor in no uncertain terms, "Sir, do not ever call me a liar again, especially in front of my classmates."

Robert soon started an after-hours job at the blood bank of the medical college. Often called out at all hours of the night, he matched and cross-matched blood for patients needing urgent transfusions. He became the blood bank czar, keeping track of when fellow students gave blood and not allowing anyone to give blood any sooner than prescribed — which often upset financially strapped students. During the summer following his freshman year of medical school, he took a job as an orderly in the operating room where Abbot worked. He mopped floors and gathered laundry, but whenever possible he could be found in one of the ORs peering over the shoulders of the surgeons. Robert dreamed of becoming a surgeon, but he and Abbot thought he would barely get through the cost of medical school; four more years of a surgery residency seemed too ambitious.

The summer following his second year of medical school, Robert convinced the operating room supervisor that he would make an excellent surgical technician — or "scrub nurse," as they were called. Thus, he spent a rewarding summer scrubbing with the surgeons on surgical procedures ranging from minor operations to major cancer surgeries. He particularly enjoyed scrubbing for Dr. Robert Haggerty, the plastic surgeon from whom he learned the skill of suturing facial wounds without leaving a visible scar. Every night he told Abbot some interesting tale about that day's surgery. Using two of Robert's favorite expressions to describe his joy in his learning experiences, Abbot said, "He was in hog heaven" and "happy as a pig in the sunshine."

Intending to learn as much as one man could possibly learn in four years of medical school, Robert attended every specialty conference he could manage, with orthopedic conferences being his favorite. He also attended every morbidity and mortality conference that he could work into his schedule.

During the summer following his third year of medical school, Robert worked at Clarendon Memorial Hospital in his hometown of Manning. Abbot and the children remained in Charleston so she could retain her job, but drove to Manning every Friday afternoon to spend the weekend at her parents' home. Robert had a room in the hospital, but he spent what few hours of the night he wasn't in the emergency room with Abbot and the children.

Upon returning to medical school in the fall of 1959, Robert savored every experience on the hospital wards, including a job at Roper Hospital sitting with critically ill patients. Dr. Larry Heavrin, Robert's fellow classmate and now a retired family physician in Spartanburg, South Carolina, remembered a dramatic incident occurring about this time in Robert's life:

Robert was interested in all of the different services that we rotated through, but seemed particularly gifted in surgery and adult medicine. One time during our junior year while he was serving on pediatrics, there was a child who had a cardiac arrest. Treatment at that time consisted of opening the chest and massaging the heart. Although there was a pediatric resident on the floor at the time, the resident was not aggressive or brave enough to open the child's chest, but Robert Jackson, as a junior medical student, went ahead and got the child's chest open and massaged the child's heart and reestablished the cardiac rate. This characterized his entire medical career in not only recognizing situations for what they were but taking care of them immediately and appropriately.

Dr. Mac Davis from Spartanburg was a year behind Robert in medical school. He knew about the above event because he and his wife ate supper with Abbot and Robert that same night:

Your dad was still trembling with the excitement of opening the child's chest and massaging his heart, which saved his life until a surgery could be arranged. He walked down the hall to the surgical suite, all the while massaging the child's heart. Afterwards, he didn't have the courage to face the family in order to retrieve his white lab coat which, incidentally, was covered in the patient's blood. Although he had just accomplished something amazing, he just unassumingly left the hospital and walked home, calling it a day. Your father's exploits spread like wildfire through the hospital, and he immediately became the hero of all the medical students.

Abbot said, "I almost fainted when Robert told me this story. I gasped and asked him, 'What if the patient had died? You would have been in serious trouble.'"

Robert replied calmly, "He was dead unless I did something. I couldn't stand by and let him die!"

Robert graduated with honors from the Medical College of South Carolina at Charleston on June 1, 1961. It was a glorious occasion for Robert and Abbot and the Jackson family. These two high school sweethearts — married at an early age, without adequate finances, bearing two children lickety-split, and despite everyone's doubts — had overcome all the odds against them and made it through not just college, but medical school as well, and with high honors at that. Who would have believed it? Even though she was eight months pregnant with their third child, Abbot cleaned and decorated their carriage house on Ashley Avenue and prepared a picnic lunch for Robert's entire extended family, her family, and some close family friends. Everyone brought something to add to the picnic, and they all celebrated Robert's graduation.

Scheduled to begin a rotating internship on July 1, Robert convinced the powers that be to allow him to begin earlier — in June rather than July — because he considered a month off to be a gross waste of time. Therefore, he actually served a thirteen-month internship. Robert entered this phase of training with his usual enthusiasm, loving emergency room duty most of all — even though, at that time, the interns worked twelve hours on and twelve hours off. Of course, Robert slept most of his twelve off hours. Abbot said of this period, "I would have been quite peeved with Robert sleeping so much had I not been so busy with our new baby John Reed, born June 23, 1961, and my new job as secretary in the anesthesiology department at Roper Hospital."

During his residency, Robert needed to decide upon a course of action to fulfill an obligation he had to the government for financial assistance for medical school. His choices: serving two years in the armed forces, or working for the Public Health Service in an underserved area of the country. He applied to the Public Health Service and received an assignment to Zuni, New Mexico, embracing it with his usual eagerness as he thought about learning new things while working with the Zuni Indians in an isolated area of New Mexico. However, the death of Dr. Scott Harvin, one of Manning's older and most beloved physicians, prompted a change in his plans. Because Manning desperately needed another physician and was classified as an underserved area, Robert returned to his own hometown as payment for his financial obligation, transferring the Public Health Service assignment from New Mexico to his beloved home of Manning, where he set up a private family medicine practice in July 1962.

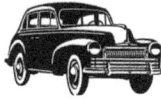

8

THE COUNTRY DOCTOR

On Wednesday July 4, 1962 (yes, July 4, per his office ledger, although a newspaper article says he opened officially on July 9), Robert's childhood dream came true — taking care of patients with medical needs in his own hometown. He opened his medical practice in Manning on Breedin Street in a small, white house with the living room converted into a waiting room and the three bedrooms into exam rooms. On that first day, his brother Scott arose before daybreak in order to be the first patient in the door. Robert saw six private patients — the last one being his brother Ralph, who he admitted into the hospital for chest pain. He saw six patients the second day — one being Ralph in the hospital; and two on the third day — one in the ER and one in his office. He even saw five patients on the first Saturday, July 7. (Reminds me of my first year when I straddled a ladder-back chair, looked out the window, and wondered if any more patients would come. I suspect we both did a lot of praying our first year. I had to see fifteen patients a day just to pay my expenses.) The next week the number averaged ten to twelve patients per day. By the end of the year, Dad cared for about twenty-five to thirty a day.

The ledger shows he charged a total of twenty-four dollars on the first day for his six patients and received thirteen dollars. Initially, Abbot was his only "employee," and Robert carried out all of the nursing, lab and medical responsibilities. He later hired Pauline Bradham as his first nurse. When Abbot had her fourth child, Richard, he also hired a part-time receptionist in the afternoon, Peggy Sue Richburg, who at that time was still a high school senior and came to work in the afternoons after school.

He became quite busy immediately — seeing patients at the office, making rounds at the hospital, delivering babies, seeing patients in the ER, and making house calls. Dad's genuine love and concern for his patients caused them to love him in return — contributing to the growth of his practice, until he did the work of two or three doctors. Nevertheless, he loved it and was, as always, "happy as a pig in the sunshine." In fact, the busier he was, the happier he was. Periodically, he took a break from the mental strain of his medical practice by attending medical meetings out of town, often planning to stay four or five days. Despite his need for diversion, he always came home a day early because he couldn't avoid worrying about whether his patients were receiving the treatment they needed.

I once heard my mom say Dad was the epitome of a caring family physician prior to also telling the story of having dinner with a young, first-year family medicine resident. The resident commented, "When I begin my medical practice, I will only see a certain number of patients per day, and when closing time comes, no one else will be seen that day."

With his ire already aroused, Dad quickly asked him, "What will you do if a distraught mother arrives with a child running a high fever at closing time?"

The young man replied, "That's not my problem."

Mom saw crimson creeping up Dad's neck, and she kicked him under the table to remind him they were in a restaurant and a "sermon was not in order."

Despite the covert warning, Dad quietly and sternly voiced his point of view. That young resident dropped to "zero" on Dad's opinion scale.

My mom continued, "I never knew your dad to refuse to see a sick child. He saw many a child in the family room of our home while we waited impatiently for that promised movie or other family outing. I have fetched many teaspoons for him to use as a tongue depressor and cleaned up many 'accidents' by nauseated children."

Somehow, the fact that Dad had a miniature medical exam room in our home on Brockington Street became common knowledge to all of his patients. The room was adjacent to the kitchen where we ate family meals. It contained all sorts of emergency and medical supplies and even an exam table. When our family arrived home from church, a long line of automobiles often stretched down the driveway, down the street, and around the corner. My mom was none too happy. Dad just smiled. These were his patients, his extended family!

Once, he counted the cars — eight total. Halfway through Sunday dinner, a tap was heard on the garage door right beside the dinner table. Mom opened the door; we all could hear an impatient but polite voice say, "How much longer will y'all's lunch be? It's powerful hot sitting out here in this car."

Robert jumped up immediately, assuring his patient, saying, "Ms. Thelma, don't you worry yourself. I'm coming right this very minute." He kindly escorted her to his in-house exam room and set about checking her over.

Well, I'm here to tell you that arrangement did not last very long. As kind and understanding as my mom is, she put a swift ending to Sunday afternoon office hours — in our house, no less!

Before Dad moved from his first office on Breedin Street to his new office next to the hospital on Hospital Street, he had me cutting grass there as soon as I obtained my driver's license. In fact, I was required to cut grass at our home, his office, and at our family lake house, plus pull all the weeds at all three locations. I wasn't all that happy about it, but I knew there was no future in grumbling. If I did, he started with the lecture of how he grew up poor on the farm, had to work hard, plowed behind a mule, and didn't have a pot to pee in. I had that lecture down pat. All my cousins had heard the same "hard luck" lecture from their parents as well. I know because we laughed about it at family reunions. Anyway, I knew better than to complain. I just cut the grass and kept my mouth shut.

One stinking hot Saturday afternoon in July after I finished cutting grass at his office on Breedin Street, I loaded the big red Toro mower (you know, the kind with the big, round bicycle tires on the back) in the rear of my mom's Country Squire station wagon. I sat behind the steering wheel for a moment, looked at all the sand in Dad's unpaved parking lot, and I don't know what really came over me. I guess I envisioned myself as a demolition derby driver. I hauled the steering wheel over to the right as far as it would go and stomped on the gas. That Country Squire had a 390-cc engine, and it jumped like a drag racer, throwing sand in a giant circle as I cut doughnuts in his parking lot. I heard the mower slam to one side in the rear, but it was too late. I was committed. After about six doughnuts, the dust spiraled in a vortex reaching up to the highest heaven. That's when I caught a shiny reflection out of the corner of my eye. I let off the gas just in time to see my dad pull into the parking lot real slow-like. The wagon jerked to a stop and rocked back and forth as heavy dust fell like rain on my car and his. Our eyes met, and he just shook his head slowly back and forth. I knew I was in a heap of trouble when suddenly two more cars pulled into the parking lot. *Ah-ha — I was saved — patients!* He slowly unlocked the back door and went inside — all the while staring me down through his bushy eyebrows like a big, angry bulldog. I nodded nonchalantly at his patients and drove off slowly like this was normal behavior for teenage boys on Saturday afternoons. He never said a word about it. I guarantee he did the same thing when he was a teenager!

Dad's pastor, Dr. Paul Sullivan at First Baptist Church Manning, wrote:

> Robert was, without doubt, one of the most competent and skilled physicians in the entire state of South Carolina. He was a man with an uncanny ability as a diagnostician, who could come immediately to grips with the physical problems of his patients, almost as if he recognized that behind his medical ability there

was the unseen hand of the Great Physician, the Lord Jesus Christ, whom he recognized and whom he served. I was honored at times to be invited by Robert to visit patients who had emotional and spiritual needs, thinking that together we may be able to help his patients. It made no difference to Robert whether his patients were white or black, rich or poor, as long as there was a physical or spiritual need. Regardless of their situation, Robert cared for them compassionately. I often saw him bow in prayer with families, but he also wanted a pastor to be there because of the spiritual credibility carried by the pastor who represents the Lord Jesus to men. I was extremely honored when he invited me to participate.

I realize that the 1960s was a time of racial tension in the United States due to the civil rights protests and desegregation, but my siblings and I were insulated from all of that because there was not a prejudicial bone in my parents' bodies. They both loved and respected the black folks who were a part of our lives, teaching us the same values. My dad's medical-practice patient population mirrored the demographics of our county, which was 70 percent African-American. I never heard him once say anything unkind or prejudicial about his black patients. More than that, when I worked in his office, I quickly came to realize that his black patients loved and respected him in return. I am convinced that racism is a matter of the individual heart that can only be expunged by the grace of God and the influence of Holy Spirit in our lives. My siblings and I are forever grateful for the example set by our parents in loving all people of all races and all social classes.

When Dad returned from Southeast Asia, he built an office by the hospital with a full lab and X-ray. His was the first medical clinic in the county to have lab and X-ray capability.

One of his first employees was Kermit Holliday. Kermit shared with me the following story:

One Sunday morning in 1971 before making his rounds, Dr. Jackson came into the lab at Clarendon Memorial Hospital. A stop by the lab was not unusual for him, but the motive that morning was a bit strange. Doc told me he wanted me to turn in my two-week notice on Monday morning because I was coming to work for him. We had never discussed this, but, being Doc, he was pretty sure of himself. He stopped back by the lab after his rounds, and the rest is history. Thus began the best seven years of my employed life. Doc was an excellent employer, and working for him was phenomenal. He told us repeatedly that his objective was to "cover Clarendon County with quality health care like the dew covers Dixie." My responsibility was the lab and the X-ray department.

One morning, I had just gotten a patient, G.L., positioned on the table for an X-ray of his lumbar spine when Doc called me to help with another patient. I told Mr. L. to just lie still, and I would be right back. When I returned in just a few minutes, he was nowhere to be found. The entire staff, including Dr. Jackson, searched the office over but could not find Mr. L. Perplexed, I went back into X-ray and found that he had somehow fallen off the table and was comfortably nestled between the table and the wall, none the worse for the experience and completely unperturbed.

I always considered Dr. Jackson an excellent diagnostician. One day, parents brought their little girl in. Doc went in the room and came out in just a few minutes and told one of the nurses to get MUSC on the phone; he needed to speak with a specialist on Reyes Syndrome. The doctor that he spoke with told him emphatically that it was impossible for him to make that diagnosis with just an office visit. After a brief discussion, the MUSC doctor agreed to see the child, and he would check her out. Eventually, he called back to the office to inform Doc that his diagnosis was correct.

Doc also took great pride in his work. He had expertise that other family doctors did not possess because of his experiences in Southeast Asia. Mr. L.B. was putting air in a lock-rim tire and the lock-rim blew off, fracturing his wrist. When I X-rayed the wrist, the X-rays revealed a real mess. Doc asked me what I thought, and I told him this was a job for the orthopedist. He studied the X-ray for a while, and finally said, "We can fix it." After anesthetizing his wrist, he went to work on it — twisting, turning, and pulling the bones back into place. Re-X-raying, more manipulating, re-X-raying, a third manipulation and the puzzle was complete. The wrist healed with 100 percent function.

Doc was also very serious about professionalism around his patients. We had a patient come in with a rectal abscess on one occasion. I got the patient prepped, and Doc came in to lance it. When the scalpel touched the abscess, it actually exploded. You really could not imagine the stench. I nearly lost my composure and said, "Oh, my God."

We finished the procedure and Doc said, "I want to see you in my office." That was the only chewing-out I ever got. Then he told me if I ever saw or heard him do anything like that, he wanted me to kick his butt.

I said, "OK."

Well, about a week later, we had another patient with the same problem. Guess who lost it that time! When the procedure was over, I said very seriously, "Doc, I need to see you in your office."

A lady from Miami was in an automobile accident on US 301. She was taken by ambulance to the ER at Clarendon Memorial Hospital. Doc was on call, so he went over to the ER to see her and had her brought over to the office. She insisted that she had to have a plastic surgeon. Doc explained that we did not have a plastic surgeon in town, and she had to have the laceration closed before the wound margins began to swell. She reluctantly agreed. Doc took pictures of the lady's face after closing all of the lacerations. A week or so later, he got a call from the plastic surgeon in Miami, who commended him for the great job he had done and said there would be almost no scarring.

There was also levity. One morning, Dr. Jackson and I were standing in the back talking when a patient, O.S., came up to us and told us we looked so much alike she had a hard time telling us apart. I assured her that it was easy because I was the good-looking one. Then she said that she wanted to see me that day because Doc hadn't been doing her any good. Doc didn't think that was nearly as funny as the rest of us did.

Another lab tech/medical technologist, Anna Lynn Floyd, a Jackson first cousin and also Dad's employee, told these stories:

Uncle Robert was more than just an uncle. He was my boss and my doctor as well — and, most of all, a good friend. When I remember him as "Dr. Jackson," I see his smiling face as he bounced into the back door of his office every morning. He never failed to greet all of his employees and patients with a cheerful "good morning."

Uncle Robert loved all of his patients and treated them with respect. In him, I saw a gentle, compassionate doctor doing his best at all times. His matchless skills, along with his particular personality, made him an exceptional physician. His talent as a surgeon, even though he was a family doctor, was unlimited. He could perform many minor surgical procedures in our office and in our emergency room. I will always remember him saying, "Cut it close to the knot" when I was cutting sutures for him. His hands seemed to glide back and forth without pausing.

A week hardly ever passed that he didn't call an office meeting.

At these meetings, he displayed some of his best attributes — loving concern and genuine affection for all people everywhere. He told us repeatedly, "Our business is taking care of sick people, and that must come first."

Some of the patients were very, very dramatic. A.D. came in with chest pain, whooping and hollering, and just really putting on a show. We put her in our emergency room in the back of the office, and Dr. Bowling, a short-term partner in Dr. Jackson's office, examined her. Dr. Jackson walked by, saw all of the commotion, and stuck his head in to see what was going on. When he saw it was A.D., he said, "Hang in there, A.D.," and kept walking by. She was instantly cured. After that, any time a patient came in putting on a show, one of us would say, "Hang in there, A.D."

Having spoken with most of the girls who were there during those seven years, I think I am speaking for all of us when I say we worked really hard, but we had a lot of fun. There was no better place to work and no better or more generous employer. It was not uncommon for Doc to bounce in the office any morning and tell our bookkeeper, Jerry Phillips, to write us a bonus check. He told us that he would not be able to do what he did if he didn't have us, and he wanted to share it with us.

My sister, Anne, recalled:

Daddy was always so energetic, and he could not tolerate laziness. He almost ran from one exam room to the next in his office, trying to keep up with the influx of his patients. When making rounds at the hospital, he took such quick strides that those of us with him had to almost run to keep up. When we asked one of the medical students who worked with Dad during the summer months how he was getting along, he responded, "My biggest problem is just keeping up with your dad."

Daddy possessed great compassion for his patients. He provided moral support during their illnesses as well as medical care. When he placed his hand on their shoulder, it let them know how much he cared, and it meant so much to the patients. It was always so touching to see how some of his patients looked up at him with such faith from their hospital beds. Hanging over the mantle in Daddy's consultation room was a well-known painting of an old doctor experiencing a night-long vigil sitting beside a sick child's bed. That painting revealed the compassion Daddy had for his patients, and we all knew that if he had lived at the time when there were no hospitals, Daddy would have spent many nights beside a child's bed.

It was my privilege to work in his office the summer before my second year of medical school. I remember his daily habit at 10:00 a.m. when he ate two chocolate-covered Graham crackers and drank two ounces of Pepsi. I observed him coming out of exam rooms, putting his leg on the stool in the lab, and writing on a chart on his thigh. All of his chart-keeping was kept on a five-by-seven index card. I never could read any of his scribble and told him so one day, to which he responded, "I'm not writing to you, Son. It's for me."

His patients would look at me and say, "Son, if you'll be half as good a doctor as your father is, you will be fine." If I heard it once, I heard it a dozen times.

I followed him through the hospital many times that summer, and, like everyone else, I had to run to keep up with his rapid and long strides. The nurses always smiled as soon as he arrived in the ER or on the floor. It was obvious they were glad to see him, and he was just as glad to see them. They were all part of his extended medical family.

Ms. Pat Newman, one of the head nurses in the ER, wrote a letter to my mom, including the following:

He is sorely missed. I miss his charm, his wit, his compassion, his knowledge, his experience, his progressiveness, and his ability to act in any given crisis. I miss his favorite quip every morning before making rounds — "OK, Pat, you got your pad and pencil? Let's go troop the line" — a saying he picked up while in the Air Force. I miss the warmth in the eyes of a patient who had suffered a stroke and had lost his speech as he listened intently to his physician as he slowly explained what had happened. He let his doctor know that he understood with his eyes and nodded his head at what his method of treatment was going to be. Dr. Jackson's pat on his shoulder always left this gentleman with a slight, drooped grin on his lips. I miss the devotion in the elderly lady's face with the malignancy as she reached for his hand when he approached her bedside. I miss his hardy laugh as she blushed when he told her how pretty she looked that morning. She quietly remarked to me as he left her room, "Lord, I sure does love my doctor." I miss his gentleness and patience as he talked with a young mother in labor with her first child, giving his reassurance as he explained everything that was going to happen. Again, his little pat on her shoulder always brought a smile to her face, no matter how painful her contractions were. I also miss his interest in tourists who were stricken with an illness while traveling through our area. Many a time I have heard him call his wife to come out and pick up a family and take care of their needs while the patient remained in the hospital.

On one occasion, my dad brought a gentleman to our home who was dressed in full military uniform and had been involved in an automobile accident with his family. He had a patch on one eye and one artificial limb. It was none other than Clebe McClary, who was slated to speak at an evangelistic crusade at the local high school that evening. My dad had cared for him and the family in the local emergency room in Manning. With both of them being Vietnam vets, they struck up a quick friendship — and Clebe, with his family, spent the remainder of the afternoon at our home with him and my dad exchanging war stories. I have to say it was a fascinating afternoon. I have seen Clebe three times over the years at various events, and each time he quickly recognized me and immediately asked about my mom. Do I really look and sound that much like my dad?

I was in the exam room one day when Dad wrote a prescription for an expensive new medication for one of his elderly female patients. When he handed it to her, she immediately responded, "Dr. Jackson, you know I can't afford that medication."

He looked at her for a moment and then said, "How much did it cost you last time?"

After she told him, he leaned over on his stool, pulled out his wallet, and gave her enough cash to pay for the medication for three months. Then he said, "We'll talk about it again at your next visit."

My sister, Anne, said:

Daddy liked to call himself the "country doctor." The name did fit him as far as his location and his close rapport with his patients — but not with his knowledge of modern medicine and techniques. He kept up with all the newest developments and was always pushing for new equipment to improve the hospital in Manning. His last big project was to create a coronary care unit and intensive care unit at the hospital in Manning. If the unit were built, he understood it would mean more work for him because he would be taking care of seriously ill patients himself rather than referring them to another, larger hospital. He sincerely wanted this because he could then offer better care for his patients. He often felt it would be better to keep his patients in Manning rather than risking a trip to another hospital, but he didn't have the facilities to care for them.

Daddy was a very capable physician and exuded confidence. This confidence caused others to place a great deal of faith in him. I recall an occasion when I made a trip to the emergency room with him. As soon as he walked in the door, a very distressed nurse shouted, "There's Dr. Jackson," and I could hear the obvious relief in her voice. I also visited the home of a family who had just lost a loved one in a tragic accident. Every person there was in a state of hysteria, and when Dad walked into the room, someone said, "Here's Dr. Jackson," with relief and faith that he would help the family in some way. The emotional chaos immediately disappeared. Dad's competence and confidence enabled him to handle many emergency situations that left other people paralyzed. He jumped into emergency situations knowing exactly what he had to do.

There was occasional excitement — like the time the phone rang and it was his brother Carl calling from the farm. Carl was breathless and his voice was barely audible. "Doc, I need help. I plowed up a hornet's nest. I've been stung at least ten times or more. You know how allergic I am. I can barely breathe."

Robert quizzed him quickly, "Do you have your EpiPen?"

Breathless, Carl responded, "Yeah, but I can't think straight. I really don't know how to do the thing." His voice trailed off and then it was gone.

Robert shouted into the phone, "Carl, Carl," but there was no response. He slammed the phone down and ran immediately out the back door. He jumped into his Pontiac Grand Prix, and in less than ten minutes he had covered the seven miles out to the Jackson farm. When he arrived, Carl was inside the big house, pale and cyanotic and barely breathing. The EpiPen was lying on the floor beside him, unused. Robert immediately plunged the EpiPen into his thigh and pushed in the medication. He began to do CPR on his very own brother, afraid that he might have arrived entirely too late — but in just a few moments' time, Carl began to breathe and his color began to return. He awakened, recovering completely. That was one bit of excitement no one cared to remember. (Remember, I told you that the Boy Scout from Sammy Swamp would years later rescue one of his own brothers.)

The following account was found in my father's files. For brevity's sake and ease of understanding, I am summarizing his typewritten report, which he entitled "Stab Wound of the Heart." (He may have submitted this to a medical journal, although this was not noted on the document.)

On Saturday, July 10, a twenty-two-year-old Caucasian male was stabbed in the chest with a steak knife with an eight-inch blade. He was able to walk to his car but could not drive due to increasing weakness. His companions brought him to the emergency room at Clarendon Memorial. Upon his arrival, his blood pressure was unobtainable and he was cyanotic. A very small wound entrance in his left lower chest was noted. IV fluids were started. Blood was cross-matched, and the patient was prepared for surgery.

The entrance wound was in the lower margin of the left lateral chest directly overlying the spleen. A wound of the spleen was suspected with accompanying severe intra-abdominal bleeding. An abdominal tap produced a small amount of blood. Chest X-ray was normal.

A left upper quadrant oblique incision was made into the abdominal cavity. To the surprise of the operating physicians, no trauma or bleeding was present in the abdomen. The patient's condition was still critical with no blood pressure. No heartbeat could be felt through the diaphragm, and immediately a suspicion of cardiac tamponade was entertained.

The left chest was opened with an incision through the fifth intercostal space. A needle was inserted through the pericardium.

A copious amount of blood was found in the pericardial sac. The pericardial sac was distended tremendously by a large volume of blood. A laceration of the heart was then suspected. The sac was opened and a large amount of blood was released. At that moment a bright, red torrent was noticed being ejected from the inferior lateral surface of the left ventricle. There was a laceration of the myocardium approximately three-fourths of an inch in length. The heartbeat immediately became vigorous again after the pericardium was opened. The wound to the heart was temporarily [staunched] by the use of two fingers while sutures were applied times two layers. The pericardium was then sutured and the chest was closed.

This case was managed in a small rural hospital by a local surgeon and a family doctor. The local surgeon had not opened a chest in twenty-five years. It was a dramatic few moments in the operating room while the heart was being repaired, but, fortunately, all events turned out well for the patient. To be able to repair a wound to the heart in a rural hospital with the survival of the patient is not an everyday occurrence in our neck of the woods. This sort of case makes one humble and at the same time proud to be a physician.

♦   ♦   ♦   ♦   ♦

William McDonald, staff writer for *The State* newspaper, wrote the following article "Rural Doctor's Day is Not a 9-to-5 Deal" on April 20, 1969:

Robert E. Jackson, MD, runs his newly renovated office with brisk efficiency. Time demands it. On an average day, he sees between fifty to sixty patients.

"You'd like to have time to talk more with your patients, but you don't. There just aren't enough doctors in town," he commented.

The doctor's office day begins precisely at 9:00 a.m. By the time he arrives at work, his reception rooms are already crowded. He hurriedly slips into the white jacket, which his nurse has thoughtfully handed him, and begins another day — which might find him working well past midnight.

9:00 a.m. — A man, middle-aged, complains of chest pain. The former patient at a TB hospital says he's been coughing a lot lately. "Now listen to me," the doctor tells him in no-nonsense tones. "I want you to have an X-ray made. When was the last time you had an X-ray taken?"

The patient, lean and with a trace of gray in his hair, sheepishly admits it's been about two years. "I just haven't had time, Doctor. I got eight head (children) at home."

9:30 a.m. — Louise, an eighty-year-old black woman and a devoted fan of the doctor's, brings in her granddaughter, age four. The girl has swollen tonsils and is suffering from a slight cold. Dr. Jackson teases Louise, whom he characterizes later as "tough." It is obvious there is a bond of affection between the two. Dr. Jackson said he "discovered" Louise living in an old tar paper shack near a fishing hole. The shack was heated by a small stove, under which is hidden her forty-five-year-old son's medicine. Her son, Levander, is epileptic and retarded. When Dr. Jackson left for a two-year stint in the Air Force, no one was sadder about his leave-taking than Louise. As she recalls, "Tears just poured down my face. I just kneeled down on that floor in there and cried."

9:45 a.m. — The doctor takes a rare break. He asks his receptionist, Peggy Sue, to pour him a cup of the soft drink he keeps on supply in the refrigerator. Dr. Jackson is concerned about a patient in the hospital, a young Marine from Parris Island, who was injured in a car/truck collision the night before. "I believe he might be psychotic," he remarked. "Physically, he's all right, but he's completely disoriented."

10:00 a.m. — A young mother comes in holding a blood-soaked cloth over her child's forehead. Between sobs, she explains that the child fell down her back-porch steps and cut his head. "Your son is not even crying, but you are," the nurse admonishes. The psychology works temporarily. A few moments later, the sobbing is renewed. "Now cut out the crying," the doctor says. "Every time you cry, the baby cries." The doctor began sewing up the child's wound, which is about an inch wide and a quarter of an inch deep. The young mother looks away and bites her lips. Tears tumble down her cheeks.

2:00 p.m. — After lunch, the doctor stops by the hospital to check on the young Marine. He says he feels a little better, but he still doesn't remember anything about the wreck. "What happened?" he asked the doctor. "A log truck hit you," the doctor answers. "Real groovy," the Marine replies. Dr. Jackson asks a few routine questions, testing further the soldier's mental condition. The answers are coherent, although a little slow. "He's done a 180-degree turn," the doctor says afterward. "I'm real pleased with his condition."

2:30 p.m. — The next stop is the farm home of Eunice, an eighty-two-year-old woman who broke her arm during a recent fall. Eunice complains a little about the pain and tells the doctor she needs some more pills for her "sweet diabetes." After examining Eunice and prescribing medicine, the doctor tells her he will see her again next month. Eunice whines, "Doctor, you mean I ain't going to see you for a month?" Dr. Jackson smiles and pats her on the arm. "I'll be back next week," he says. Before leaving, the doctor participates in an old custom still observed by some of the residents in the rural county. Almost ritually, he washes his hands in a pan of water placed atop a wood stove along with a dry towel. "If I didn't wash my hands after a visit, they would be offended," he smiled.

8:00 p.m. — The doctor is a guest speaker at the Kingstree Lions Club. He talks about his experiences in Southeast Asia and shows slides of some of the wounded he treated. Some slides are so gruesome that one of the members becomes visibly shaken.

12:30 a.m. — The doctor checks by the hospital for any emergency calls. As no calls have come in during his absence, he decided to call it a day. "It's a rat race," he reflected on the drive home. "No, it's not a rat race," he replied after a brief pause. "You've just got to have the right attitude. If you don't have it, you might as well throw in the sponge."

3:00 a.m. — The doctor receives an emergency call. A middle-aged man had been brought to the hospital suffering from severe facial wounds.

Such was the life of the rural family doctor in the '70s.

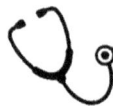

9

HOUSE CALLS

"**H**ello! This is Dr. Jackson."

"Dr. Jackson, this is John R. You know my foreman F.M. Well, his wife has been in labor for over twelve hours now. The midwife just called me and said I needed to call you immediately. There seems to be some problem with her labor."

Dr. Jackson questioned, "Did she specify what the problem was?"

"No sir, she did not. She just urged me to call you and say it was urgent."

Robert's attitude about medical practice was that he should serve the people. He was always ready to make a house call no matter how far into the country he had to travel.

On this occasion, he had to drive to the far corner of Clarendon County during a heavy rainstorm. Mr. John had to drive him up to the wood-frame house in his pickup truck because the rain had flooded the yard. Robert jumped from the truck onto the porch and went inside to find a house full of children, a distraught father, and a mother in hard labor. He examined the mother and found it would be a short while until she delivered. He reassured the father and the midwife, then sat in a rocking chair beside a blazing fire with the father until the midwife called to say, "It a-comin', Doc, it a-comin'." The delivery was soon accomplished successfully.

Once my mother rode with Dad, as she often did just so she could talk with him and be with him. The autumn weather had turned unseasonably cold, as dry yellow and red leaves propelled by the wind danced across the paved roads of Clarendon County. Driving slowly down a long, sandy dirt road, they arrived at a small, unpainted wood frame house nestled in a wood lot that was surrounded by vast fields of golden, uncut soybeans. As her husband, the country doctor, parked right beside the house and stepped on the porch of the rickety, two-room house, Mom jokingly said to him, "If you need any help, just call!"

About ten minutes later, he beckoned for her to come inside. Swallowing hard and regretting her offer to help, she dutifully entered the house to find that Dad had delivered twins. They were so tiny, he could hold one baby in each of his hands. He handed one baby to Mom, with instructions to take him to the car until he could tidy up, so they could take the baby to the hospital for special care. Mom thinks this twin died while in the hospital, but the tender care and concern that she observed her husband providing to the mother and the babies touched her deeply. Mom never forgot this perfect demonstration of her husband's love for each one of his patients and how each was special to him in some way. She said, "He felt honored to be chosen to treat his patients and was always willing to become involved in their problems, whether medical or personal."

The things that happened to him on house calls were often so bizarre they did not require any hyperbole — like the time he took my brother John Reed with him on a house call out in the country when J.R. was in elementary school. They decided to drive the little yellow Triumph Spitfire that Dad had purchased for my mom. It was a delightful two-seater with a four-cylinder engine and four in the floor. It was a particularly pretty day in the fall of the year. Dad was fond of wearing a tan newsboy cap when driving the Spitfire for style and to prevent the wind from blowing his hair.

John Reed traveled with our dad to a farmhouse set off the main road about a quarter of a mile. When he had completed his house call, Dad jumped over the side of the Spitfire into his seat without opening the door since the convertible top was down. He gave one of his famous grins, fired the engine up, and put it into first gear. Suddenly out of nowhere, a really big dog with a giant head came bounding toward the little car, giving out a deep-throated bark. He was twice as tall as the little Spitfire, and his face was covered in slobber. Dad let off the clutch, and the Spitfire bogged down momentarily in the deep sand, making John Reed's heart jump into his throat before the little car shot forward in a slewing, sideways motion, throwing sand out behind. The dog was on them in an instant with his big, slobbering head right beside Dad, barking at full volume. Dad slid as far over toward John Reed as he could. He continued to work the gears until they outpaced the snarling dog. They both stared at each other wide-eyed, and John Reed realized the left side of Dad's face was covered in dog slobber. Dad gave a nervous laugh and slid back into his seat; then they both began to laugh like little girls for several miles. Just another story for Dad's doctor bag!

Then there was the time … "Dr. Jackson, this is Mr. E. Me and Mama went to the state fair in Columbia today and walked a 'fer piece' all day long. Now I'm bleeding somewhere, and I can't seem to find the spot. Do you mind coming to the house and checking me out?"

"Mr. E., I'll be right out there."

In another fifteen minutes, Robert pulled up in Mr. E.'s driveway and walked up on the porch. Mr. E. and his wife were in their late seventies, and both were hard of hearing. Robert knocked loudly on the door twice and got no answer. He opened the front door, stood in the wide breezeway constructed down the middle of the old antebellum home, and announced his presence. Still no answer. He walked in a few more steps, and there on his left was Mr. E. — stark raving naked with his giant, obese abdomen out in front, straddling a mirror on the floor trying to observe from where he was bleeding. About that time, he shouted to his wife in the next room, "Mama, my belly has done got so big, I can't see myself."

To which she responded cynically, "You ain't missing much."

Well, Robert got so tickled, he had to retreat to the front porch to give a belly laugh or two, regather his composure, and then re-enter the house to complete his house call. Turns out Mr. E. had "gaulded" the inside of his overweight thighs by walking too much in the heat at the fair. Some medicated salve and two bandages later, and Robert was on his way with another story to tell — anonymously, of course.

On another occasion, a female patient called late on a Saturday night crying with anxiety and depression, begging her doctor to pay a visit. He drove down to Santee to a lake house near the water. The patient was a big woman — maybe 280 pounds — and she was emotionally distraught. She spent some time detailing the trauma of dealing with her unruly children and losing her job. She then stood, walked to the door, and said, "Dr. Robert, I do declare it is terribly hot in here." She slid off her housecoat, exposing a sheer, see-through negligee underneath; all 280 pounds of her glory was clearly visible. As she leaned against the door, her intentions were plain. Now family doctors are accustomed to seeing women in such a state every day, but usually with bright lights in a sterile medical office and with a nurse chaperone. This spectacle in low light in her small living room — with no chaperone — and her leaning against the only escape route, wearing next to nothing but a sly grin, was quite distressing.

Dr. Robert had his wits about him. He smiled shyly, patted the couch beside him, and clutched his doctor's bag with his other hand. She took the bait and literally skipped across the room to sit on the couch beside him. As soon as she sat, Robert was up like a wild buck fleeing from a thicket. In two strides, he was out the back door with his bag in hand. "Jack be nimble, Jack be quick." In a few more steps, he was at his car shutting his door as he heard Delilah say, "Dr. Jackson, don't leave. You misunderstand me."

"Yeah, right!" It was shortly after this that he announced an end to making house calls. The official reason announced was that he could not obtain necessary labs in private homes, but we all knew better — Delilah had scared the bejeebers out of him!

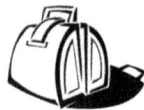

10

THE ART OF PARENTING

"Robert, I am really having difficulty with this renal physiology. Do you mind if I come over and study with you tonight?" asked the future Dr. Larry Heavrin, one of Mom and Dad's best friends in medical school who described Dad as "one of the better students" in their class. Larry studied with Dad frequently and spent many evenings reviewing class notes in my parents' apartment at Robert Mills Manor, affectionately called "the project."

After a couple of hours of studying one evening, Dad looked at me and directed, "Robin, it's time for you to go to bed. Upstairs, Buddy-boy."

I immediately put away my toys and walked upstairs to my bedroom like a good little soldier. I knew better than to protest or raise any fuss or commotion. When my dad said, "Hop," you would think you were at the Eastdale Bunny Farm. There were kids hopping all over the place!

As I walked up the stairs, Larry observed, "That's very impressive. I don't know many four-year-olds who would go to bed without any protest."

As a very strict disciplinarian, my dad expected instant obedience, an expectation he probably acquired from his own father, the father of ten children. We all came to understand this as the years passed. Balancing love and discipline in the life of a child is a delicate proposition, but I think Dad learned the balance fairly well. We respected our father, which kept us all out of trouble during those years, but we also loved him because he loved us well and disciplined us appropriately. The fear of the Lord and the fear of Dad is a good combination. Of course, children never understand discipline to be appropriate at the time, but in the end, it produces the "peaceable fruit of righteousness."

When my brothers were in high school, we attended a church Christmas play in the church's gymnasium. The bleachers had been arranged in a semi-circle around the stage at one end of the gym. About three-quarters of the way through the play, a commotion occurred among the high school students on one section of the bleachers. As it turned out, my two brothers were the instigators at the center of the commotion. Although he sat two bleachers away, Dad stood up and started pointing repeatedly at them while glaring through his thick, bushy eyebrows. One of the teenagers immediately noticed and punched my brothers. Jerking their heads up in alarm, they spied Dad pointing at them and glaring like a fierce Doberman. They immediately shut up and sat up — straight as little soldiers. The entire section of students did the same; not a peep was heard from any of them for the rest of the program. The adults all smirked with approval.

At the conclusion, Dad made a beeline for "the boys." He grabbed them by the elbows, escorted them out of the gym, placed them in the backseat of his car and took them home. They didn't pass go and they didn't collect $200; they went straight to jail. Upon our later arrival at home, the door to their bedroom was closed; we weren't sure exactly what happened, but we didn't see them again until the next morning when they arrived at the breakfast table — sullen and pouting. We all noticed the next week that they rode their bicycles everywhere they went and not in Granddaddy Jackson's old, tiny, baby blue Rambler pickup, which Dad compelled them to drive for a year to improve their humility quotient before they were allowed to acquire their own vehicle. (My uncles and older cousins derived a great deal of pleasure/humor watching the doctor's sons driving Granddaddy's baby blue Rambler truck around town.) Their conduct and their humility quotient drastically improved after this heart-to-heart discussion with Dad!

Driving home from the farm as a seventeen-year-old, I ran into a thunderstorm while driving my mother's yellow Triumph Spitfire. Thankfully, I had the convertible top up, so I avoided being drenched by the summertime downpour. However, the zip-up plastic window behind my seat was still unzipped, and rainwater blew in the window. Foolishly, I tried to zip up this window while I drove, glancing over my shoulder to do so. When I shifted back around and glanced through the windshield, to my horror my little car had completely drifted off the road onto the wide, grassy shoulder. About 100 yards in front of me was a four-by-four wooden mailbox post. I glanced at my speedometer and was again horrified to see I was going seventy miles per hour. Knowing I could not jerk the car back onto a wet road, I tried to ease it back on, but, alas, the car began to immediately spin. Two quick spins and now I was traveling backwards at seventy miles per hour on the opposite, grassy shoulder. I looked in the rearview mirror, and I could see a Volkswagen coming in my direction. The car spun one more time, crossed the road, and went nose-first into a clay bank, stopping on the side with the driver's side door down. I quickly undid my seatbelt, crawled out the passenger side door just as the car rolled over, crushing the convertible roof. I stood there in the pouring-down rain, infuriated with myself for wrecking my mom's car, and began to kick the rear tire.

The baby blue Volkswagen pulled up beside me. It was Mr. Graham, a rural mailman and the father of one of my best friends. He just looked at me sadly and reproved me, saying, "Son, you should be thankful, not angry." Then he offered to take me home to the lake house. I went in the house and sat on my bed, soaking wet and dreading my dad's appearance. I knew he would see the upside-down car on his way home from work. Sure enough, about fifteen minutes later, I heard his car come roaring into the driveway, throwing gravel against the metal storage building. Soon after, I heard his feet pounding into the house and down the hallway. Dread filled my soul!

Immediately, he called out, "Son, are you all right?"

Fearing the worst, I replied meekly, "Yes, sir. I am fine. I'm sorry about the car. Are you mad at me?"

"Son, don't worry about the car. I can replace it, but I can't replace you." He put his arms around my shoulders and immediately began to pray over me, thanking God for my safety. The wise preacher in Ecclesiastes said, "There is an appropriate time for everything. And there is a time for every event under heaven." I realize there is a time for rebuking a child, and then there is also a time to refrain. Dad wisely spoke the right words for this moment in my life, and I have never forgotten them.

When Dad was in his medical residency program in Charleston, South Carolina, our family attended First Baptist Church of Charleston. Although only six years old at the time, I recall the experience vividly. Dr. Hamrick was pastor at that time, and I recollect him being tall and dignified. Of course, as a six-year-old, I don't remember a word he ever preached, but I am certain that the Word did not return empty or void but was planted in fertile soil.

What I do remember most clearly were the squeaky doors at the end of each pew. If you've ever been to First Baptist Church of Charleston, you would have seen the little white wooden doors affixed to either end of each pew, as was customary in many churches built in the early 1800s. Now rather than paying attention to the sermon, my little mind was fascinated by the challenge of opening that door without making it squeak, which, of course, would disturb the polite silence of the auditorium and bring annoyed glances from adults.

On one particular Sunday morning, my mother made the mistake of allowing me to sit beside the door. I kept eyeing the door until I couldn't withstand the temptation any longer. *Could I push that door open slowly enough that it would not squeak? Would it not be a major triumph if I could get it all the way open without the hinges making the slightest noise?*

Slowly, ever so slowly, I surreptitiously pushed that door with my little sneaky hand. A loud squeak of the hinges penetrated the respectful silence. I jerked my hand back as my mom reached over and pinched the pure-tee-living-fire out of my thigh. I bit my lip and forced myself not to cry out. After all, I had six-year-old friends in the service, and I had a reputation to uphold.

Well, foolishness is bound up in the heart of a child. I'm fairly certain there was a pickup load of foolishness bound up in my heart at that time because I kept eyeing that door. Sure enough, I tried once again to win bragging rights in the six-year-old boys' Sunday School class. As I pushed that door ever so slowly again, it squealed like fresh tires on new asphalt!

In a flash, my dad jerked me up by the arm and lifted me over the squeaky door, and down the aisle we went — with all of my horrified friends watching aghast. There was no rod of discipline to drive the foolishness out of my heart. He simply applied the flat of his palm to my bare thigh twice in rapid succession right there on the front steps of First Baptist Church, in front of God and every tourist walking by gazing at the historic building. Then he stood up straight and tall and pretended he didn't even know me. I began to caterwaul like my pet collie did when he got a treble hook caught in his front paw. He sat on his haunches, held up his front paw, and commenced this high-pitched squalling. I was performing a close imitation when my dad leaned over and said, "Dry it up, boy, or I'll give you something to really cry about." Shoot dog, I already knew what that meant, so I dried it up quick like. He hauled me back down the aisle, still snubbing, to the approving smiles of the adults and the apprehension of my peers.

I had the keen foresight to position my mother between me and the squeaky door. I didn't even look at that door for the rest of my life. Once burned, twice shy.

All manner of squeaky doors exist in our lives that we shouldn't sit by, touch, or even look at. You know what they are in your life. If you aren't certain, ask Holy Spirit. That's His ministry — to clarify for you the source of temptation in your life. I would like to say I have been as successful in my adult life at staying away from squeaky doors as I was for the rest of our stay at First Baptist Church, Charleston — but that wouldn't be truthful, and you would know that. Sadly, for me, my Heavenly Father has had to discipline me on multiple occasions for messing with other squeaky doors.

You know the temptations/squeaky doors in your life. Just don't sit next to them. Don't look at them. Don't touch them. Squeaky doors come in different shapes, sizes, and colors — so does temptation. Put the Word of God between you and the squeaky door, and don't even look at it. When my sibs and I were growing up, our mother said to us repeatedly, "A word to the wise is sufficient."

'Nuff said.

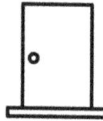

11

BEST DAD EVER

Dad shouted to me, "All right, run ten yards, fake right, and cut across the middle. I'll hit you as soon as you turn to the left. Be ready."

In the fall of the year, Daddy always pretended to be Terry Bradshaw of the Pittsburgh Steelers, his favorite quarterback. I was Lynn Swann, his favorite receiver. Just about every afternoon after work, he threw me passes as he worked on his throwing game, and I worked on my receiving. The only problem: I was as slow as Christmas. I mean, like a water spigot: I ran a long time in one place. That didn't matter to Dad. He just needed a receiver. I was available and I could catch his bullet passes.

The same thing occurred in spring and summer. I played first base and had this long, floppy first baseman's glove that I loved dearly. It was like a vacuum cleaner. It sucked up everything he tossed my way. He intentionally threw balls at my feet or over my head for hours on end, or so it seemed to me. He always encouraged me and told me how great I could be. It stood me in good stead for my high school baseball years when my third baseman and shortstop threw the ball wildly in my direction. I was used to it by then. Surprised by my ability to scoop up throws in the dirt, my high school baseball coach asked, "Where did you learn to catch like that?" Thinking nothing of it, I shrugged and said, "My dad coached me."

My JV football team headed to Kingstree, South Carolina, one Thursday afternoon, which happened to be my dad's afternoon off. It was pouring down rain when we left Manning and continued to rain heavily throughout the ballgame. Because of the rain, the only people present were the players, coaches, and cheerleaders. The downpour soaked everyone completely within seconds of getting off the bus. Thankfully, it was a hot August day, so no one was really bothered by the rain. Playing football in the rain was just another adventure to us teenagers.

I have no recollection of who won that football game, but here is what I do remember. At the end of the fourth quarter, I remember being called to the sideline when a sub came in to replace me. The rain fell so hard we could barely see the sideline from the middle of the field. As I jogged off the field, I heard the JV cheerleaders calling out, "Two bits, four bits, six bits a dollar. All for the Monarchs, stand up and holler." There was only one fan in the stands, clothed in a long raincoat and holding an umbrella; he stood up and hollered. As I looked closer, it was my dad — the only person in the stands for either team. As you can imagine, this scene left a never-ending impression on my mind — but not just mine. Twenty years later, one of the cheerleaders came up to me and said, "You remember that game in Kingstree when it was raining so hard, and we cheered and your dad was the only one in the stands?" Yes, I will always remember.

When we were young, Dad had an imaginary friend named Joe who had all kinds of adventures. After supper each night, his friend Joe called on the phone from somewhere in the world, often the Grand Canyon, and told Dad about his misadventures — like falling off his donkey and down the side of the canyon. Dad repeated the stories to us kids while holding a spoon up to his ear as if it were his telephone. Entirely caught up in telling the tale, he would start laughing until tears rolled down his cheeks. The more he laughed, the more we laughed. Then the stories would become more and more outrageous!

I sat in Mrs. Barnes' fourth-grade class, cutting up with my fellow classmates one day, when my friend Freddie tapped me on the shoulder and pointed to the back of the class. I looked back, and, to my shock, there was my dad with that stern expression of his that made grown men tremble. What business did he have in my school building in the middle of the week at 2:00 in the afternoon? Heaven only knows, but he caught me red-handed. He pointed his finger at me and mouthed the words, "Come here." He grabbed me by the scruff of the neck and hurried me to the little boys' room and wore my hind end off. It was humiliating, to say the least. I returned to my seat, sat down and trembled like a little pup. I kept looking over my shoulder, but he was gone. Word got out and everyone in my class and three other classes knew exactly what happened to me that day. My dad's appearance terrified everyone on that hall, and to the teachers' delight, it also produced well-behaved children for weeks on end. We all kept glancing nervously at the back of the classroom for a long time, wondering if he might reappear. As for me, I'll tell you God's truth — I never cut up in that fourth-grade class again. I was constantly looking over my shoulder. In the small town of Manning, my dad seemed to be omnipresent — and he had spies everywhere. Like I said, the fear of God and the fear of Dad is a great combination that contributes to well-behaved children!

I discovered later that the high school principal had called his office to say, "Doc, we have your high school ring here at the office. Can you come by to pick it up?"

Dad responded, "That's impossible. I lost that ring during high school while swimming in Black River over in Kingstree." It seems that he and his friends were swimming in Black River one hot summer day when he lost the ring, never to be found again — or so he thought. Eleven years later, a dredging company had been hired to remove mud from a section of the river when his ring was discovered in one of the pump's filters. The foreman cleaned the green ionization off the ring, read the school name and initials inside the ring, and contacted Manning High School. After consulting the yearbook for the class of 1954, my dad's initials were the only ones to match. As he retrieved his long-lost ring, he happened by my fourth-grade class and instilled the fear of Dad more deeply into my little renegade heart!

My brother Richard talks about Dad's love for golf and for our mom:

When we were in junior high school, Dad took all of us boys to play golf after church quite frequently during the summer months. Dad was so much better than we boys, but he took his shot and waited patiently while we attempted to hit the ball as far as he could. Between the three of us, we lost a hundred golf balls while Dad patiently watched, usually laughing under his breath. Before he hit his drive at the tee box, he looked down range, squared up to the ball, waggled his hips, and then before his back stroke, he always said, "Ride 'em, cowboy." Then he knocked the cover off the ball.

As teenagers, J.R. and I were rather silly, making noises right before he tried to tee off. As a serious golfer, this initially made him rather angry, but when he looked around, he saw his three sons smiling and laughing at him like three monkeys. What could he do? He wasn't going to spank us in a public place, so all he could do was laugh. It only got worse after that. He never knew when he could tee off before one of us would make an unexpected sound. It really drove him crazy, but it drove us to tears. Those were great days.

One of my best memories was watching Dad hold Mama's hand at the dinner table and looking at her with so much affection in his eyes. We could all tell he really loved our mom. I heard a preacher say once that the best gift a man can give his children is to love their mother. Well, we were blessed because our dad sure loved our mom.

My brother John Reed recalls Dad's teasing:

When we were just little tykes, we loved for Dad to scare the wee willies out of us. He would hide somewhere in the house, turn out the lights, and wait for us to find him. When we found him, he emerged with a loud roar, and we scattered throughout the house, screaming and knocking things over. On one occasion, he sent Richard and me to our bedroom for bedtime. Shortly thereafter, we heard a scratching at our window and opened the blinds to find Dad outside with his face pressed against the window, shining a flashlight under his chin. With his face contorted, he scared us half to death. We jumped up in the middle of our bed, hugged each other, ran in a circle, and then took off running out of the bedroom, but on the way out a big hairy arm reached out of the closet and grabbed us. We both fell on the floor, still running in place. The arm belonged to big brother Robin. They had planned this venture together, and they got what they wanted — two seriously scared little boys. Afterwards, the two of them went to their bedrooms, and we could hear them laughing for a half hour afterwards. We heard our mother say, "You shouldn't scare my babies like that." Trembling, Richard piped up and said, "Yeah, you shouldn't scare her babies like that." Ever after that event, big brother Robin could walk by the door of our bedroom and throw a pair of rolled up socks across our bedroom against the blind on that window, causing the blind to automatically roll up, terrifying us all over again. Our dad and our big brother were terrorists long before terrorism was popular.

Once upon a time, we found a baby squirrel and were nursing it to health. We enjoyed playing with it for several days until one morning we awoke to find it had died. Dad was about to leave for work when I came into the house, holding it in my hand and informing him that it had died. I was probably only about eight years old at the time, and I was grief-stricken. He sat me down and put his arm around my shoulder, explaining, "Sometimes these things happen, even when we try our best." He had such a commanding personality and was such a take-charge kind of guy, but at times he could be so kind and sensitive. This revealed a side to him I had not seen before.

Dad constantly gave us chores to do around our house — chores like emptying trash, cutting grass, pulling weeds. Of course, we never wanted to do any of these things, so we were perpetually complaining. His response was always: "You boys don't know how good you have it." Looking back on it, I realize we slept right up until time to go to school in the morning, and then after school we took a nap right up until ball practice. On the weekends, we hung out with our buddies, doing pretty much whatever we wanted to do. Then we complained about cutting grass with a riding lawn mower. When I was older, I realized I complained to a father who had to feed chickens and slop hogs before school in the morning, and who had to plow behind a mule after school before doing his homework in the evenings. Upon reflection, I realized he was right. We really didn't know how good we had it.

Richard and I were the least studious students in our entire high school, which caused much chagrin for Mom and Dad. Every night after supper, Dad asked us if we had homework to do. We usually hemmed and hawed around before he sent us to our bedroom to do our studying, but we listened to music and played around. Rarely did we study.

On one occasion, Dad burst into our room, and, with a stern expression, demanded, "Have you boys been studying?" We both jumped about a foot off our beds. We then stared at each other for a second, then looked back at Dad. Richard replied, "We're fixing to get ready to start thinking about studying." Dad stared at us perplexed for a moment, and then he shook his head and said, "I don't know what I'm going to do with you boys" — his standard expression of exasperation. That response became a classic still used in our family to get a good laugh. I feel certain he learned it from his father, who raised eight boys.

Once, Mom and Dad had a party at our house. We ended up misbehaving badly. Dad had all he could stand of us, and sent us to our bedroom and told us to wait for him. We heard them joking and laughing for what seemed like hours down on their end of the house while we waited on our "executioner" to finally arrive. We sat on the edge of our beds, nervously rubbing our thighs and looking at each other with big, wide eyes. Finally, he came abruptly into our bedroom, scaring us so badly we jumped off our beds. It must have been comical, because he burst out laughing, began shaking his head, and said, "I don't know what I'm going to do with you boys." He then left the room as abruptly as he came. Looking at each other in surprise, we heaved a big sigh of relief.

My sister, Anne, remembers:

When we were older teenagers and in our college years, Sunday night after church became a special family time. Mom cooked scrambled eggs, grits, and bacon for supper. We ate until we were full, often fighting over the last biscuits. Then we sat around the table, talking or telling stories of our childhood. We teased each other in good fun. We often had friends over who enjoyed our family times as much or more than we did. Dad often pushed his very thick eyebrows to the middle, where they stuck hideously straight out, making us all laugh even more.

John Reed continues:

Dad was always a man of integrity. He often carried us to Clemson football games on Saturdays, which was always a source of great delight for us. We flew up in his airplane, taking only fifty-five minutes compared to a four-hour road trip. At one of the Clemson football games we attended, two guys seated behind us were overly rowdy and drinking alcohol. (Dad was a teetotaler and always said, "If you never drink the first drop, you'll never get drunk.") Dad asked them politely to calm down and not to curse, especially around the ladies. They paid him no attention, continuing to be overly loud and profane, at which time Dad decided we should leave. When he stood up, one of them knocked his hat off with a big foolish grin. Dad only repositioned his hat on his head and kept moving forward. We boys were always impressed with that moment as our dad could have easily taken them down in their intoxicated state, but chose the more noble path as an example for his boys.

Dad always said, "Nothing good happens after 11:00 at night," so the rule was we had to be home by 10:55 and in bed by 11:00 p.m. This particular Saturday night, I was way past curfew when I decided to take a detour down a secluded dirt road to take my girlfriend home. I got stuck — really stuck — in the mud. We had to leave the car and walk a long way to a farmhouse to ask for help. It was totally humiliating, but even more frightening to call my dad. Dad was there within twenty minutes, picking us up and driving her home without any recrimination. He was very understanding and hugged me on the way home, saying, "Let's keep this between us." Now you know why we consider him to be the best dad ever.

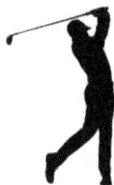

12

DOCTOR DAD

"Hey, Doc. I won't keep you but a minute. I hate to bother you on the weekend, but my hemorrhoids have been killing me. You know, swelling and bleeding. Can't go without crying like a baby. What do you think I ought to do?"

"I'm sorry, sir. This is his oldest son. He won't be home for another hour. Can I take a message?"

Embarrassed, he answered, "Oh, I'm sorry, Son. I thought you were your dad. You sound just like him. What do you think I should do?"

I guess folks thought I picked up medical school just by osmosis by living in the same house as Dr. Jackson, because I remember many such phone calls at our home as a teenager — especially when my voice began to change. Patients mistakenly thought I was my dad, so they immediately launched into a description of their medical issues. Called "Little Doc" from as early as I can remember by uncles and family friends, I wore that appellation with pride because my dad was a man of integrity, a kind and compassionate physician, and beloved by the community he served.

My siblings and I all learned how to sound professional with neat-sounding orders like, "Give 'em 50 mg of Demerol and 50 of Phenergan, and I'll be there in fifteen minutes," because we had all heard Dad say that hundreds of times over the years. We often sat around the dinner table and imitated him just to make him laugh. One of us would pick up a spoon, hold it to our ear and say with a serious expression on our face,

"Give him nitroglycerin. Get an EKG and I'll be there in five minutes." Then we all howled with laughter.

John Reed recalls, "We grew up with our dad being our family and team doctor. That was just normal for us. Oftentimes when we were injured, Dad taped us up so we could continue playing. Once in a basketball game, I ran head on into another player, which caused me to lose consciousness. Before I blacked out, I saw Dad rushing to me and realized he had caught me before I hit the floor and then carried me off the court. What a great doctor dad!

"Dad sewed up our lacerations and set our broken bones. When I broke my collarbone, it was badly out of place. Dad repositioned my collarbone once, but the first attempt was not successful. Therefore, it required a second repositioning. However, it was so very painful for me he couldn't bring himself to do it a second time, so he asked another doctor to complete the procedure. It's funny the things we remember."

◆   ◆   ◆   ◆   ◆

Richard tells this story:

One summer day at the lake, Robin asked me, "Richard, you want to go on a ride on my dirt bike?"

"Sure. Let's go!" I eagerly exclaimed, always ready to go on a bike ride.

It was one of those ninety-nine-degree, super-humid days down at Santee when we loaded up on Robin's dirt bike and began touring the sandy back roads around the lake. We rode all through the dirt roads around Santee, just cruising and having fun. At one point, I looked back, and with dismay I shouted over the roar of the dirt bike, "Robin, stop, stop! There's Rock! He's been chasing us." Unaware that Rock, our Irish setter, had followed us for several miles on that extremely hot and humid day, running the entire time, we stopped — and he fell over, exhausted, his chest heaving like a bellows and his head straight up in the air, gasping for oxygen.

"Richard, he is in serious trouble. We need to get him to Dad's office. You stay here with Rock and I'll go get John Reed and the station wagon."

In short order, we rushed Rock to Dad's office in town. We carried him in the back door and laid him on the exam table in the surgical suite. Our doctor dad appraised the situation, listened to his heart with his stethoscope, and started an IV in his hind leg. All three of us boys were scared to death. Our dad's patients must have been mystified to walk by and see a big, red, hairy dog lying on the exam table with an IV and three skinny boys rubbing his head. They probably never forgot that sight. Just another day in the life of our doctor dad.

That same dog Rock bit a fishhook at the lake house one day. It was a lure that had a treble hook at each end. He bit the lure and the hook on one end went through his lip. This startled him so much that he jumped and caught the hook on the other end in the curtain a few inches from the floor. Now trapped in the curtain, Rock began a constant, ear-splitting yelping. Mom and Anne began "freaking out." Mom ended up holding Rock while Anne cut the hook out of the curtain (that curtain had a hole in it for years after), so Dad to the rescue again. In desperation, Mom called him at the office. He left dozens of patients at his office and quickly drove the ten miles to the lake house. He got some wire cutters, and we held onto Rock while Dad cut the barbed end off and slid the rest of the hook out of his lip. Removing treble hooks from fishermen or their family members (or pets) is a regular occurrence for any family doctor within striking distance of a fishing lake like Lake Marion.

John Reed fondly remembers:

While playing golf one Sunday afternoon with Dad and my brothers, we heard an awful commotion off in the distance. We could tell it was the sound of an unhappy dog. We looked around and there came Eddie Barrett, the golf pro, and our mom dressed in a yellow pantsuit in a golf cart carrying our other Irish setter Sage in her lap. Sage was bleeding profusely from the mouth, and blood was all over Mom's yellow suit. Mom had a stricken look on her face, and Eddie wasn't too happy himself. Sage had bitten something sharp and lacerated a vessel underneath his tongue. With each heartbeat, bright red blood squirted from underneath his tongue all over Mom. Dad immediately reached into his mouth and squeezed the bottom of his tongue. We all left the back nine, put Sage back in Mom's blood-covered back car seat, and headed to Dad's office while Robin continued to apply pressure to the poor dog's tongue. Dad placed Sage on the same surgical table where Rock had once lain and went to work. He found the laceration, stopped the bleeding, and sewed up the wound. Doctor Dad to the Dog Rescue again.

My sister, Anne, says:

Daddy appreciated anything anyone did for him, and he was always quick to say how grateful he was. I worked in his office during the summer for several years and observed the relationship he had with his office staff. Many times, he held a special meeting in his consultation room just to say thank you to them. This meant a lot to the staff, and in return they were very dedicated to him. On the few times I made hospital rounds with Dad, I noticed he always thanked the hospital staff for all they did. At home, he always thanked Mama for what she did for our family. If I fixed him a little snack, he would thank me just as if I had done something really special. Because of his gratefulness, everyone was always eager to do anything for him. He, of course, liked to be appreciated for what he did, but all he wanted was a "thank you." He once gave me a yellow lollipop at his office, and I replied, "I would rather have a red one." He looked at me with a disappointed look and said, "When someone gives you something, don't complain about what color it is." That exemplified his attitude, which has always stuck with me — making me attempt to be a more appreciative person.

Daddy was an enthusiastic person and never went about anything halfheartedly. The best example of this would be his medical practice. If he was going to be a medical doctor, he was going to be the best. He was always willing to go to medical seminars to learn more so he could give better care to his patients. He always went the extra mile to be sure he was doing everything possible for them. He went about everything in his life with enthusiasm. Many times, he told us children that "if you're going to do something, do it right." Once he committed himself to doing something, he did it gladly and wholeheartedly, whether it was teaching a Sunday School class or doing something with his medical practice. This has always challenged me to do my best.

◆ ◆ ◆ ◆ ◆

One Saturday, my dad quickly walked through the den and called to me, "Robin," as I sat watching a football game on the sofa, "come on, boy. We're going to the ER." Well, my little heart skipped a beat. I was only in high school, but I already knew I wanted to go to medical school and become a family doctor like my dad. Any exposure to the ER was an adventure to me.

When we arrived, Dad tried to introduce me to one of his alcoholic patients, but the man was snoring loudly, completely intoxicated. He had fallen out of his back door at home, hit his head on the concrete steps, and split his forehead from his nose to the hairline all the way to the skull. Most of the bleeding had already stopped by the time we got there.

Dad put in a few stitches, carefully showing me how it was done. Then he had the nurse put sterile gloves on me, handed me the instruments, and said, "Go to it, boy. I'll be back after I make rounds on my patients." I smiled and pretended like I did that sort of thing every day. Inside, my heart fluttered. I sutured his forehead slowly and painstakingly for an hour, finishing up just as Dad returned. Always the encourager, he looked at my handiwork, smiled and said, "You might just be a surgeon." All the nurses laughed (probably at my suturing), but I was never happier. That was in the early '70s. I'm certain you couldn't get away with that in today's world of HIPAA regulations and liability.

During the summer of 1978, between my first and second years of medical school, I worked as an intern at Dad's office. A patient presented to his office who had dropped a chainsaw on the front of his right leg. It had glanced off the front of his shin, leaving dozens of superficial lacerations that required suturing — just what an aspiring medical student needed for practicing. The patient was agreeable after my dad explained who I was and the experience I needed to gain. He sat patiently for three hours while I sutured dozens of superficial lacerations. The practice was invaluable preparation. I recall my first rotation in the emergency room in medical school where my classmates and supervising residents stood in amazement while I sewed up lacerations with expertise, not requiring any instructions. Thanks, Dad!

Two years later, before my senior year of medical school, I water-skied at Santee with some of my medical school friends when I stepped on something sharp, lacerating the bottom of my foot. I knew immediately it would require sutures. Two of my medical school friends went with me to the emergency room in Manning. When we arrived, the emergency room overflowed with patients. One of the ER nurses recommended we come back at a later hour. She put a pressure bandage around my foot, and we left to eat supper in town. We returned about 9:00 p.m. as dusk fell on the little town of Manning and found the ER empty of patients, so I stayed. The staff registered me and told me to get up on a gurney. Shortly, a beleaguered and very irritable resident came in to evaluate my foot. Curt and somewhat rude, he was obviously not happy to see me.

I realized immediately the difference between him and my dad and how they dealt with patients. It dawned on me that this was the first time I had required any kind of medical attention since my father's death and the first time I had not seen him come bounding in with his usual energetic enthusiasm and that infectious smile on his face. The wound on my foot was nothing compared to the sadness in my heart that suddenly washed over me as I keenly felt his absence.

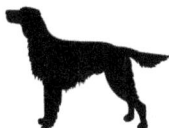

CITATION TO ACCOMPANY THE AWARD OF

THE BRONZE STAR MEDAL

TO

ROBERT E. JACKSON

Captain Robert E. Jackson distinguished himself by meritorious achievement as a Field Medical Officer while participating
in sustained medical operations in Southeast Asia from 29 July
1966 to 7 December 1966. During this period, Captain Jackson
demonstrated outstanding medical skill and courage in successfully
accomplishing medical operations under extremely hazardous conditions. On 15 August 1966, a critically wounded X-ray technician
required immediate evacuation from a take-off strip that had no
navigational aids, was closely bounded by mountains, and was ob-
scured by weather. Captain Jackson, because of his intense desire
to help a fellow man, accompanied the patient, who required constant medical attention due to his injuries, to a field hospital and
thereby saved his life. The exemplary leadership, personal endeavor, and devotion to duty displayed by Captain Jackson reflect
great credit upon himself and the United States Air Force.

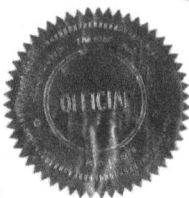

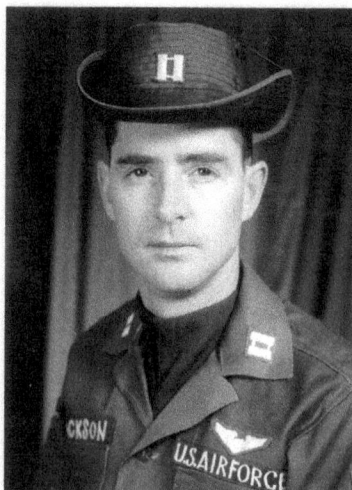

*Chapter 1 — Captain Jackson in
Air Commando uniform, which he
never wore while undercover in Laos*

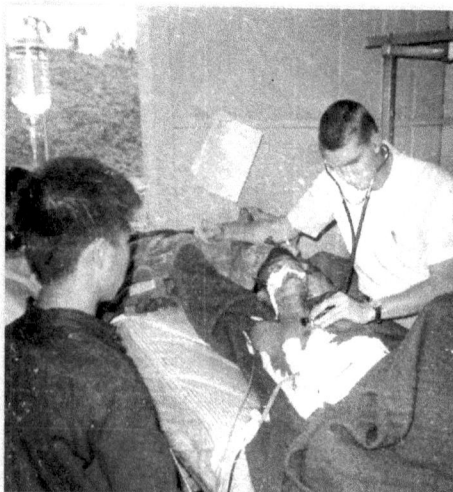

*Chapter 1 —
Examining post-op patient*

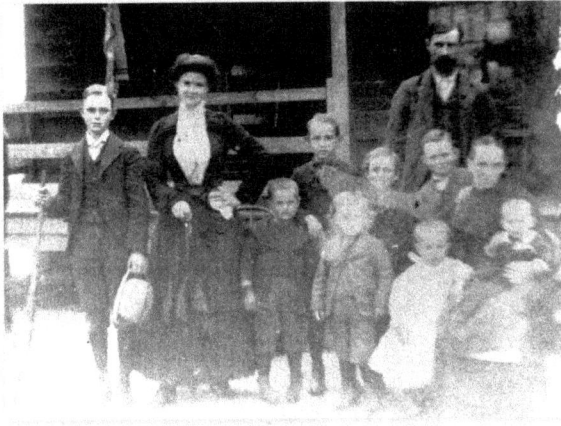

Chapter 2 —
Thomas Jehu
Jackson Family

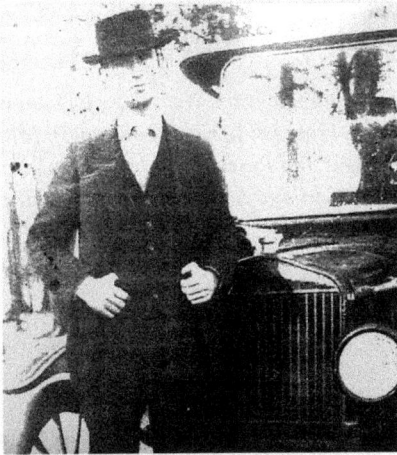

Chapter 2 —
M.R. (Moultrie Reid) as young man

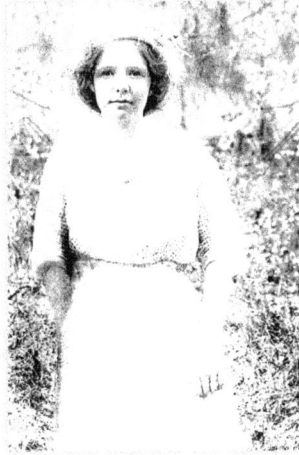

Chapter 2 —
Anna Charlotte Singleton

Chapter 2 —
"The M.R.
Jackson Home"

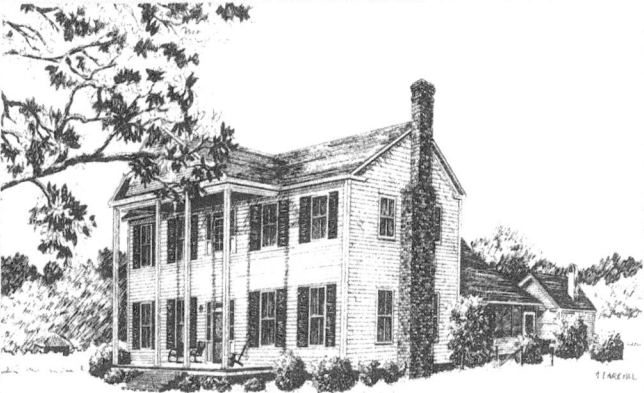

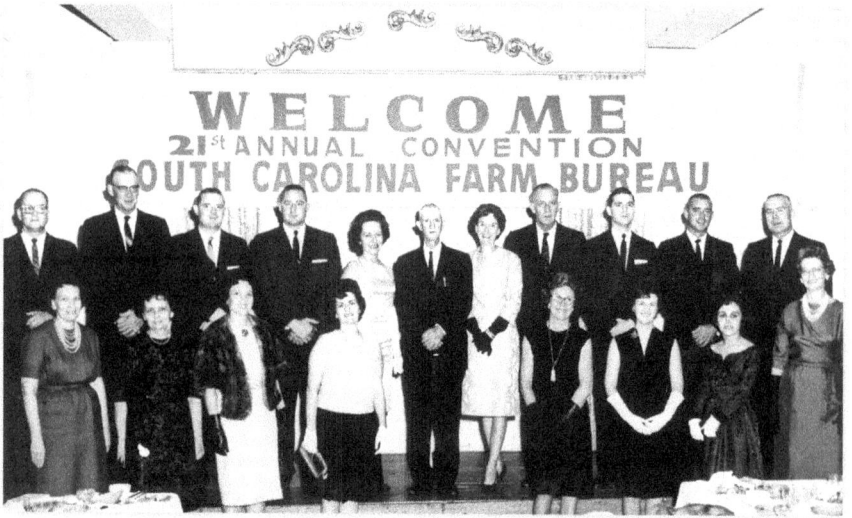

Chapter 2 — Entire family attending Farm Bureau event when Papa Jackson was honored by the South Carolina Farm Bureau. From left to right (both rows): Jehu and Julia, Billy and Laura, Ralph and Olivia, Scott and Roseanne, Edna, Papa Jackson, Eunice, M.R. and Pearl, Robert and Abbot, Carl and Margaret, Jimmy and Mary.

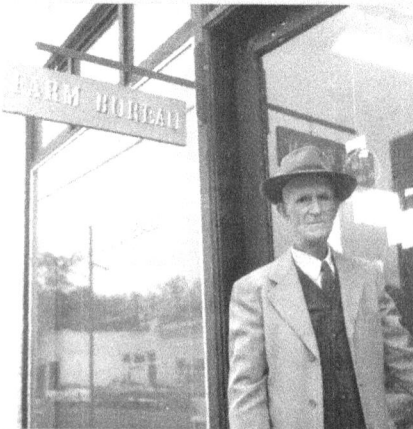

Chapter 2 — Papa Jackson standing outside Farm Bureau office

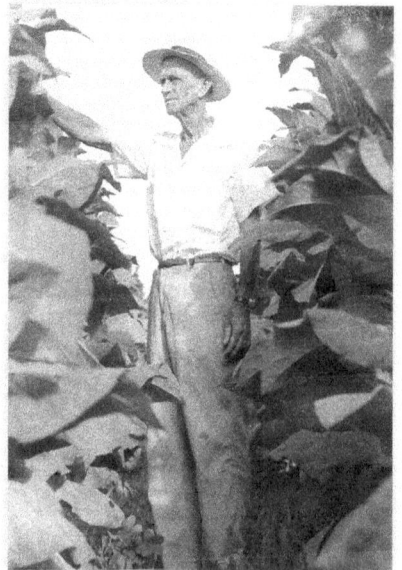

Chapter 2 — Papa Jackson in tobacco field

Manning Times

Of All: The News of Clarendon County Completely And Accurately Reported

Manning, South Carolina Wednesday, August 9, 1978   15 CENTS PER COPY   14 PAGES

Chapter 2 — Local newspaper records M.R. Jackson home on fire

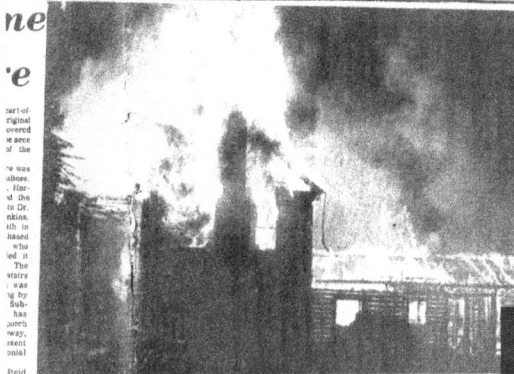

Chapter 3 — Robert's brother Scott as Clemson football player

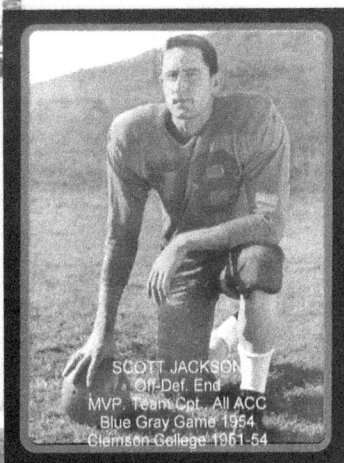

SCOTT JACKSON
Off-Def. End
MVP, Team Cpt., All ACC
Blue Gray Game 1954
Clemson College 1951-54

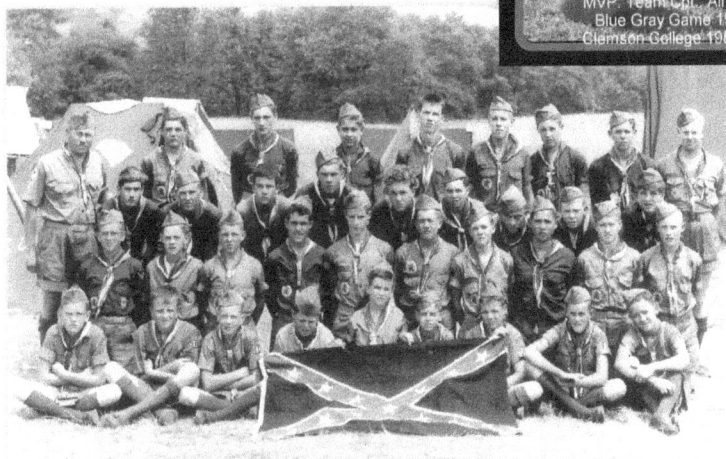

Chapter 3 — Boy Scouts of America Jamboree, Valley Forge, Pennsylvania, June 1950 — Robert Jackson, Mike's rescuer (second row from bottom, fourth from right)

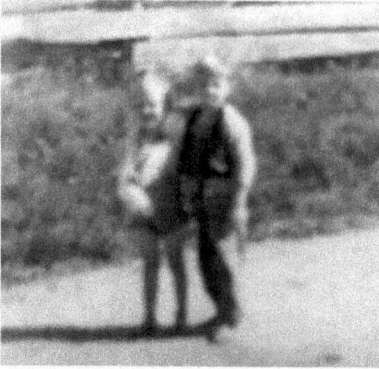

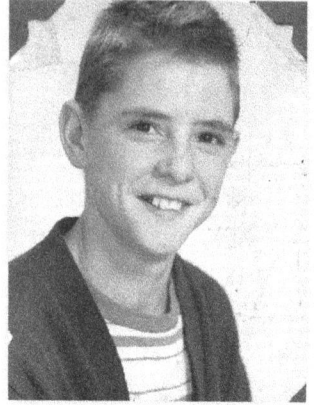

Chapter 3 — The paratroopers:
Robert (left) with arm in cast,
and Carl (right)

Chapter 3 —
Robert as a grade school boy

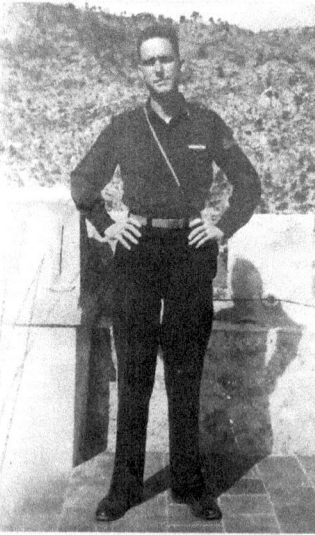

Chapter 4 —
Captain Williford
Stuckey "Jimmy"
Jackson, Bronze Star
recipient for bravery on
the battlefield, WWII

Chapter 5 —
Robert as field general

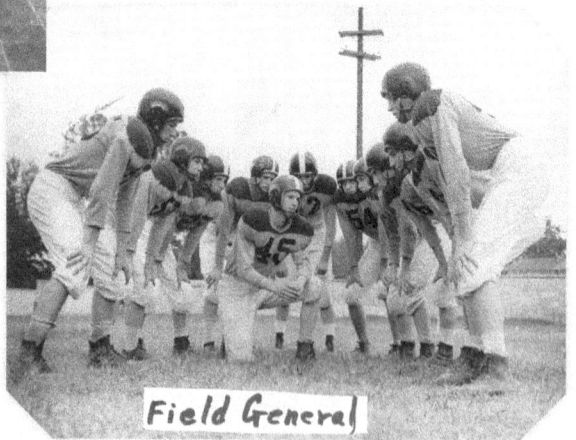

Field General

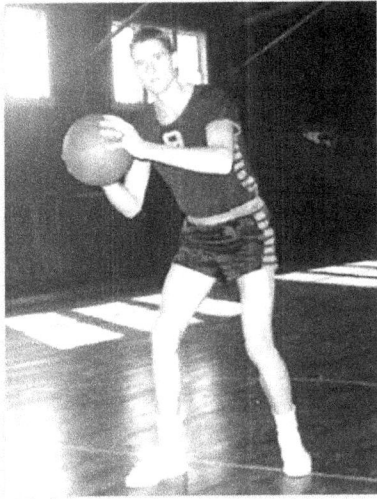

Chapter 5 — Co-captain, Manning High School basketball team

Chapter 5 — Behind the plate for Manning High and Post 15

Chapter 5 — Charleston newspaper reports on American Legion sectional meet

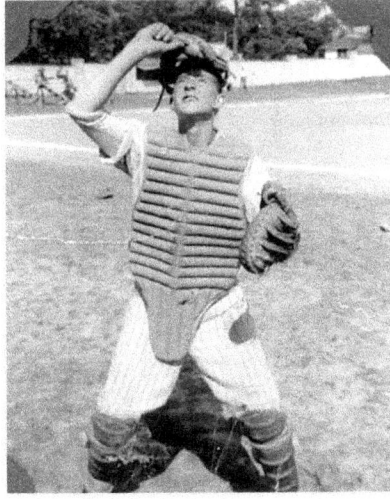

ies'

accompa-
ve in the
theastern
d Series."

The News and Courier

CHARLESTON, S. C., SUNDAY MORNING, AUGUST 24, 1952

Sumter Legion Juniors
Arrive Today
for Sectional Meet

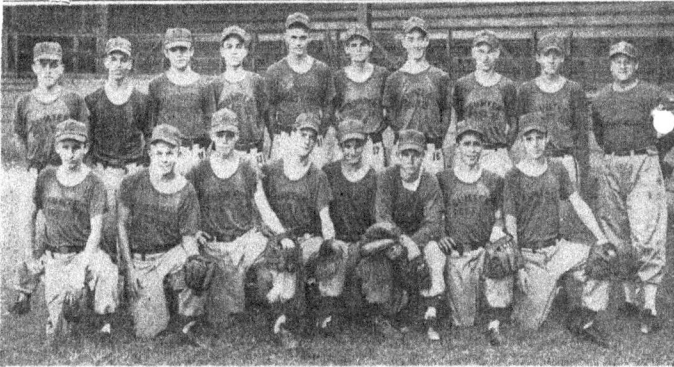

REGION 5 CHAMPS—The Sumter American Legion Junior Gamecocks who defeated Marietta, Ga. for the Region 5 title and who will play Memphis, Tenn. in the opening game of the Section B tourney here tomorrow night are pictured, left to right, front row: Billy Ray, Don Gallup, Irvin Plow- den, Robert Jackson, Jimmy McDaniel, Norwood Reardon, Alex Grubbs, and Sammy Gantt. Back row, Pat Kelly, Robert Richardson, Jack Hodge, Kenny Rosefield, Pete Gibson, Sammy Moore, Bill Kolb, Don Frierson, Clarke Watts, and Coach H. N. (Hutch) Hutchinson.

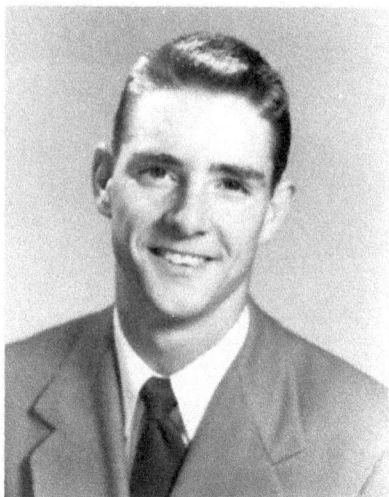

Chapter 5 — Manning High School "Boy of the Year," 1953-1954

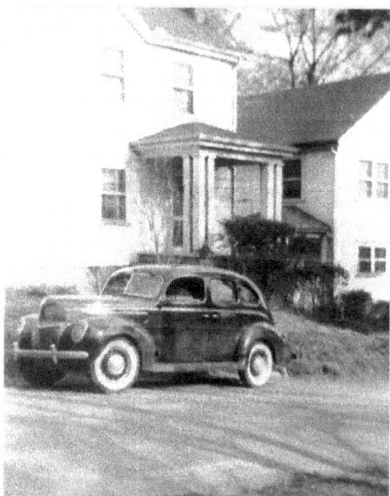

Chapter 5 — Sixteen-year-old refurbished 1939 Ford sedan driven to Clemson College

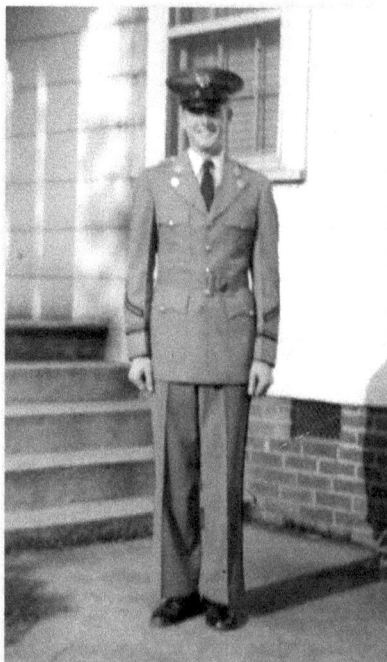

Chapter 5 — Robert as ROTC cadet at Clemson

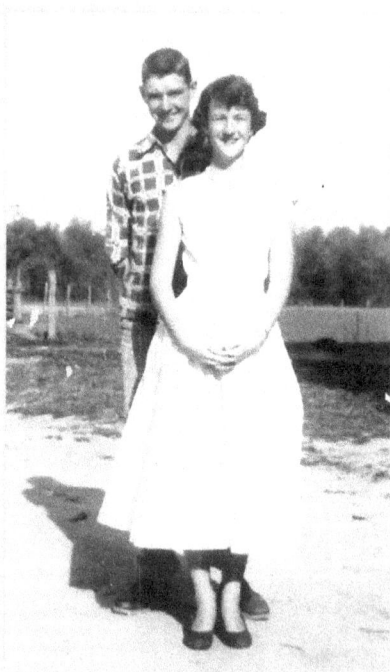

Chapter 5 — Newlyweds

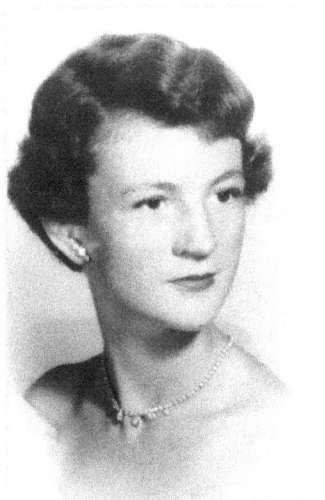

Chapter 6 — The bride
Anna Abbot Land Jackson

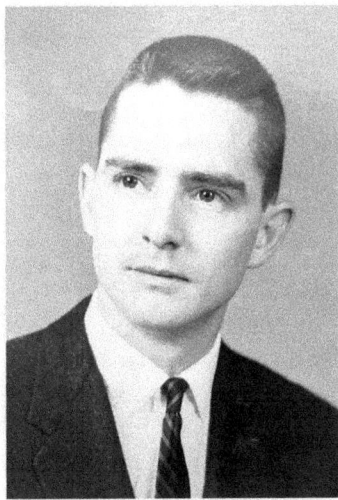

Chapter 6 — The groom
Robert Edward Jackson

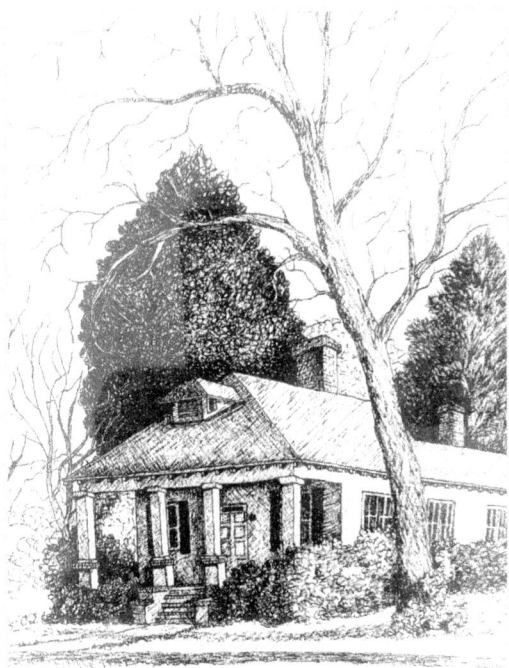

Chapter 6 —
Abbot's childhood home on Church Street

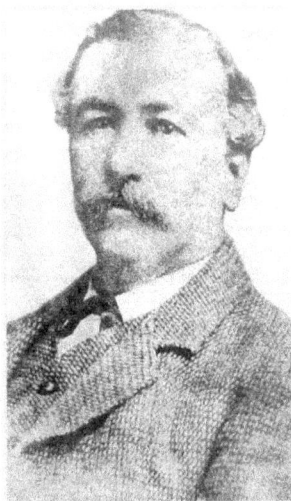

C. S. LAND (1833–1899) MUSTERED INTO
the Confederate Army as a private in
January 1861. He was promoted to
the rank of major before the war
ended. Land served continuously for
more than four years with no time off
for sick leave.

Chapter 6 —
Major Ceth Smith Land

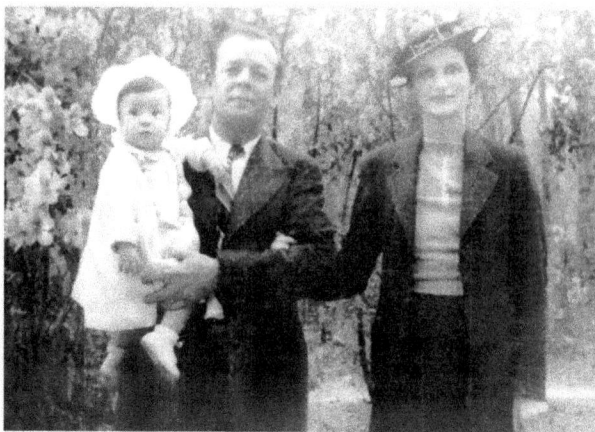

Chapter 6 — "Coon" and "Anne" Land with daughter Abbot

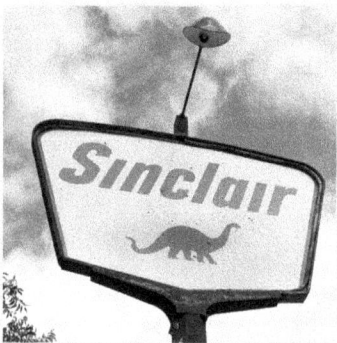

Chapter 6 — Sign like the one above "Coon" Land's gas station

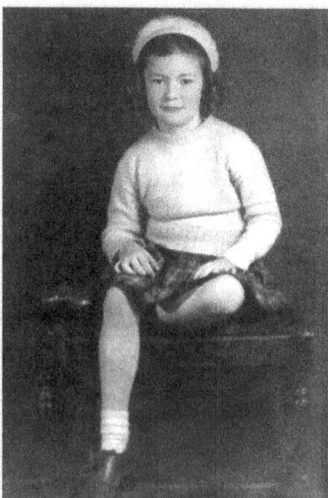

Chapter 6 — Childhood picture of Abbot

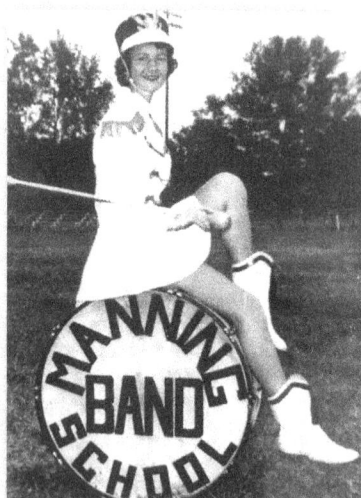

Chapter 6 — High school majorette

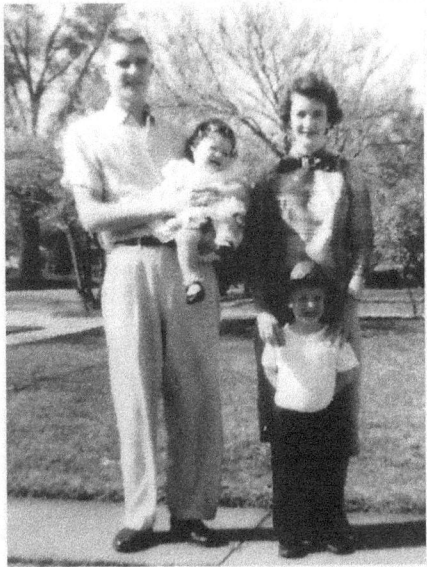

Chapter 7 — *Robert and Abbot with Robin and Anne*

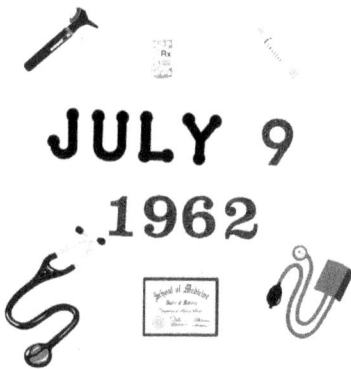

JULY 9 1962

ROBERT E. JACKSON, M. D.

ANNOUNCES THE OPENING OF HIS OFFICE
FOR THE GENERAL PRACTICE OF MEDICINE AND SURGERY

AT

208 BREEDIN STREET
MANNING, S. C.

OFFICE HOURS   TELEPHONE:
10 TO 1 AND 3 TO 5   435-9390

Chapter 8 —
Announcement of office opening

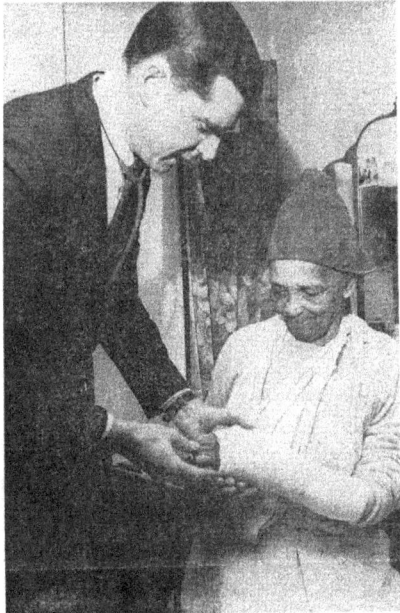

A House Call In Rural Clarendon

Chapter 8 —
House call with patient

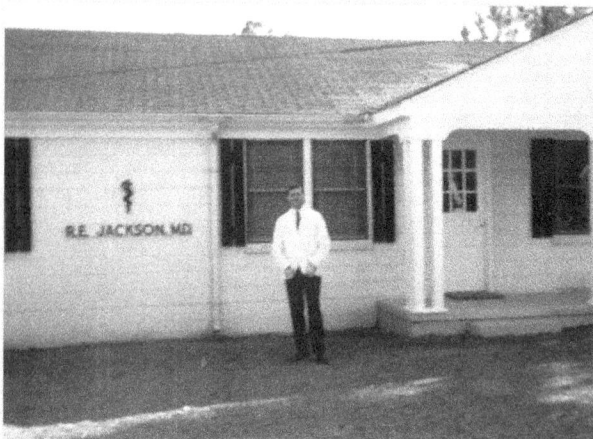

Chapter 8 —
First office on
Breedin Street

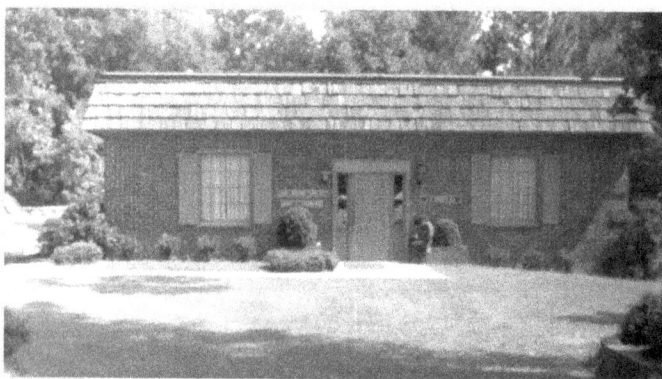

Chapter 9 —
New office on
Hospital Street

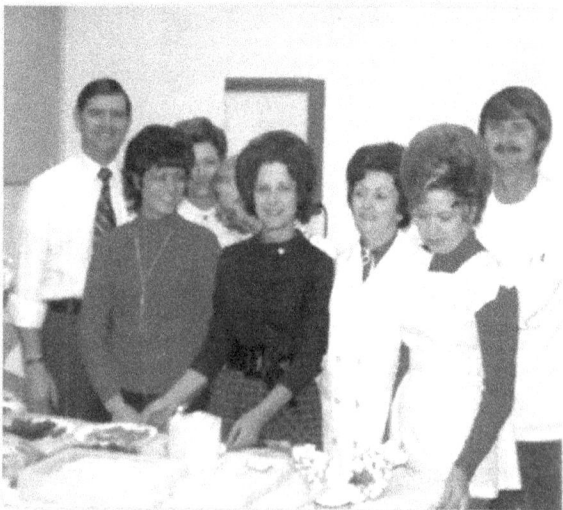

Chapter 9 —
Employees in 1972

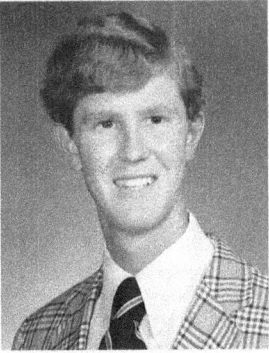

Chapter 11
Me — "Robin"

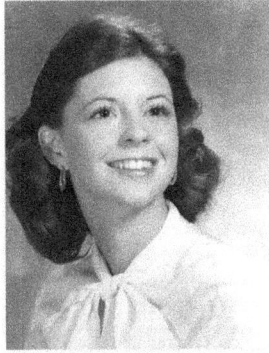

Chapter 11
Anne — "Sugar"

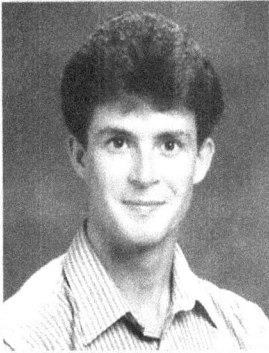

Chapter 11
John Reed — "Reedy"

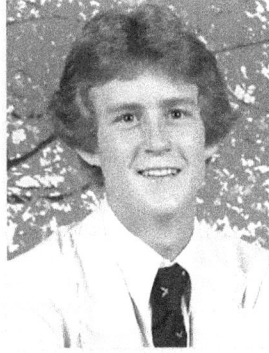

Chapter 11
Richard — "Rich"

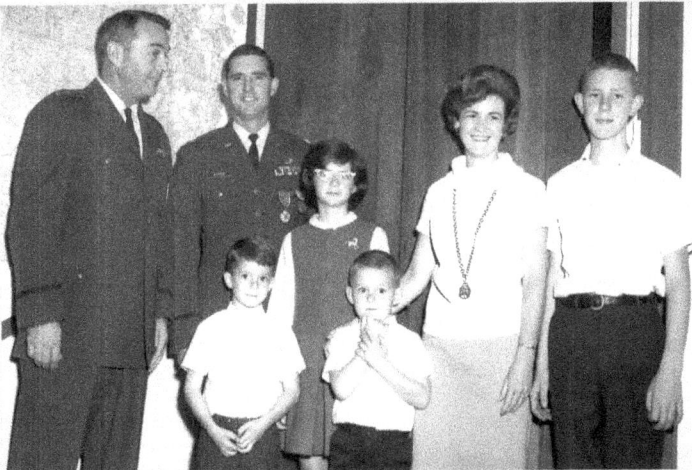

Chapter 11 — Our family

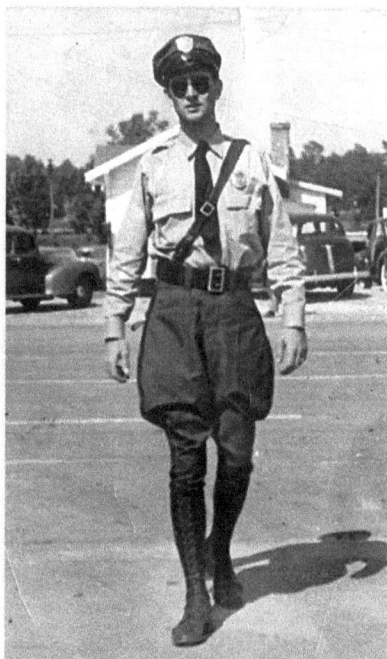

Chapter 13 — Robert's brother Jehu in highway patrolman uniform, 1940

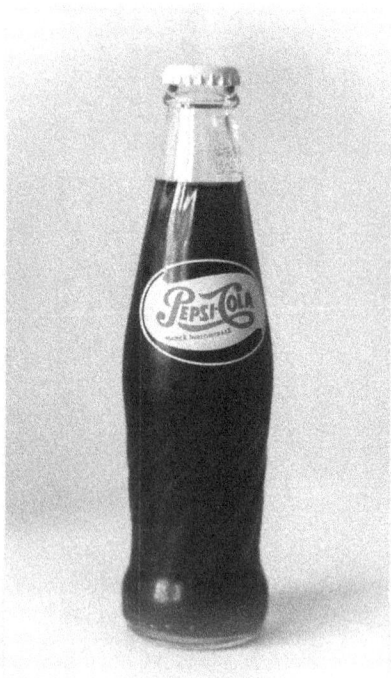

Chapter 13 — Dr. Jackson carried his own Pepsi to every party so all would know he wasn't drinking alcohol (photo courtesy of Lulia Buta, Unsplash)

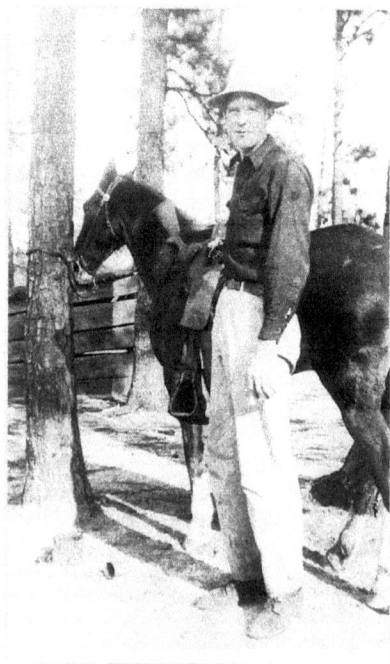

Chapter 14 — Robert's brother Billy as quail-hunting guide

13

A Strong Conviction

During Robert's youth, his second oldest brother Jehu, who was twenty years older than he, served as a highway patrolman — first for Lexington County, then for Calhoun County. He patrolled as the lone highwayman on an Indian motorcycle for a combined ten years. Transferred to Manning in 1951, he once again served as the only patrolman on a heavily traveled Highway 301 running through the middle of Clarendon County.

The highway had already become a major thoroughfare from New York to Miami before the interstate system, especially during holiday seasons. The normal two-lane traffic passing through Manning became four lanes during major holidays, because as drivers turned right on Sunset Drive (still Highway 301), the roadway widened to accommodate four-lanes of traffic. Frustrated drivers immediately tried to pass one another to gain a little advantage; however, because our town was so small, before they knew it a bottleneck occurred at the edge of town only a couple of miles further south as those four lanes transitioned back to two lanes.

My friends and I often stood on the sidewalk and talked to weary travelers as they crept along through the middle of our hometown. We laughed at their northern accents as they laughed at our southern drawls. My sister, Anne, and I — entrepreneurs that we were — made a financial killing one hot Fourth of July weekend selling lemonade off a card table for five cents a cup. I poured, and she handed it through the car windows. Many northern travelers had never seen cotton up close, so local farmers often left several rows of cotton next to the highway, allowing travelers to stop and pick a genuine southern souvenir as they traveled through the Deep South during the late fall months.

In 1952, Jehu resigned his position and ran for sheriff of Clarendon County, winning that election by a wide margin. That was the first of his seven consecutive terms — twenty-eight years as sheriff — one of the longest terms of office of any sheriff in South Carolina.

While in high school, I was driving out of town on Highway 261 late — almost at dusk — one Saturday afternoon. I looked in my rearview window and spied a blue light flashing. I couldn't imagine what I could have done wrong, but I dutifully pulled over to the side of the road and parked my car. I got out my license and my registration and just waited for the officer to walk up to my car. When he approached, the officer was none other than my uncle Jehu, the lawman. I had committed no infraction of the law. My only crime was being one of thirty-one nieces and nephews. Recognizing my automobile, he had only pulled me over to chat. We sat on the hood of my 1973 Pontiac Grand Am until it was completely dark — just chewing the fat with the blue light slowly turning the entire time.

Finally, I said, "Uncle Jehu, you've got the blue light going, and all my friends are driving by wondering what in the world I have done wrong. I think it's about time I got going."

He responded, "Would it make you feel better if I wrote you a ticket?"

I said, "No sir, I'll just be on my way."

Some years later when I was courting my future bride, Ms. Carlotta, I called Uncle Jehu and inquired about borrowing his Harley-Davidson Electra Glide, which he was more than glad to share with me. I had planned to impress my new girlfriend by taking her on a motorcycle ride to Myrtle Beach. The only problem was his bike had "Sheriff Jackson" stenciled on the tank in large block letters, and at age twenty-three, I was obviously not the sheriff of Clarendon County. He placed several layers of masking tape over his name and sent us on our way. Wouldn't you know it, before we left Clarendon County, we encountered a highway license check. The highway patrolman could see Sheriff Jackson's name clearly through the masking tape. He kept eyeing my driver's license and the sheriff's name, barely discernible, through the tape. I could see the wheels turning as he was calculating whether or not this skinny red-headed boy was really the sheriff's nephew, as I had declared, or whether I was a thief making off with the sheriff's motorcycle. He stared at me and the pretty girl on the bike and then decided he wasn't about to take a chance. He wasn't going to be the highway patrolman who allowed a young punk to make off with the sheriff's motorcycle. He went to his patrol car and made us sit in the scalding hot sun while he made a few radio calls. He returned in about fifteen minutes, smiled and nodded, and very respectfully wished us a good day. We did indeed have a good day — driving Uncle Jehu's Harley-Davidson all the way to Myrtle Beach and back.

I remember traveling with my father to Uncle Jehu's home one Saturday morning when I was in middle school. Dad was called there to care for an injured prisoner. The sheriff's home doubled as the county jail. We entered through the front door, passed through the kitchen, and then through a heavy metal door that separated the home from the jail in the back. My aunt Julia was in the kitchen preparing food for the odd assortment of prisoners present on this particular Saturday morning.

I entered with my dad and Uncle Jehu, who was wearing his sheriff's uniform, including a white starched shirt, tan pants, and a wide black belt with a pistol on one side. I remember being very impressed with how official he appeared, even though he was quite jovial and pleasant toward all of his inmates.

I sat on a wooden bench and glanced at two other disheveled men sitting on another bench across the room being processed by a deputy. They appeared none too happy and smelled of alcohol and urine. One of them had a black eye and a swollen face. They both looked my way and nodded. I didn't know whether to smile or wave, so I just nodded, trying to be cool — like I came to the jailhouse every day.

There were two cells — one for whites and one for blacks (remember, this was the '60s in the Deep South, when segregation was standard) — both containing several men. My dad seemed to have a prior acquaintance with all of these men, because as soon as he walked in he called several of them by name, and most of them said, "Hey, Doc!" Uncle Jehu opened one of the cell doors, which made me a bit nervous, but Dad walked right in without hesitation and began shaking everyone's hand as if they were dignitaries. They all stood and immediately showed him equal respect. The other men reached through the bars to shake his hand as well. Looking back on it, Dad impressed me with his immediate rapport with all of the prisoners and how friendly he was to all of them. It was obvious that he was respected by all people, regardless of their class or situation.

He tended to a man with a large swelling on the back of his head, who had been knocked unconscious in a fist fight outside of a juke joint near Davis Station. Dad looked in his eyes, made him stand on one leg and then the other, and made him answer a few questions. He then declared him safe to remain in the jailhouse. As he left, he gave him a stern warning about strong drink and being out with the wrong crowd. After the cell door closed, he looked at all of them and said, "That goes for the rest of you, too. If you stay away from booze and bars, you won't end up in the sheriff's little bungalow overnight." He smiled at them, shook hands all around, and then we left. As we drove away, he looked at me and said, "Boy, if you don't drink the first drop, you'll never get drunk."

♦   ♦   ♦   ♦   ♦

Dad always had an intense antipathy toward alcohol and its impact on his patients and their families. Many of our family weekends and holidays were interrupted by calls from the ER requesting his presence to care for alcohol-related motor vehicle accidents, domestic disputes, and personal injuries. The Clarendon County Saturday Night Knife and Gun Clubs were usually lubricated with alcohol, leading to gunshot wounds and stabbings, which required the doctor on call to investigate. Although he despised the effects of alcohol on his patients, he never seemed to lose his affection for or kindness toward them. On multiple occasions, I watched in the ER as he rebuked an intoxicated patient while tenderly and expertly suturing their lacerations, setting their broken bones, or ministering to their broken hearts, as was so often the case after domestic altercations. I am confident that the Great Physician was active in my dad's life, working through him to speak words of truth in a loving and compassionate way. His patients always seemed willing to accept an honest and hard admonition from him because they also knew he cared deeply for them. Speaking the truth in love is a delicate balance, and my dad seemed to have perfected the art.

When I was in medical school, I was on a surgical rotation with Dr. G.B. "Crow" Bradham, who was an acquaintance of my dad. Dr. Bradham was a stern, no-nonsense, physically imposing attending physician who intimidated most of the medical students and residents. He was well known for interrupting students in mid-sentence when they were making their patient presentations by asking them questions to throw them off their train of thought. He had little patience for incompetence.

One of my fellow female students had been up all night admitting patients and did not have all of her lab values together for her patient presentation. The most important lab value in a post-operative patient is the patient's hemoglobin, which she did not have that morning. She began by making excuses, saying, "I'm sorry, Dr. Bradham. I was up all night in the ER admitting multiple patients."

At this point, he put his hand in front of her face and said, "Stop! Ma'am, I know that life is tough. I just want to know what the patient's hemoglobin is." That sent shudders down the spines of all of the rest of us peons.

Once when another student was making his presentation, he caught me looking at my note cards regarding my patient. He stopped the student in mid-presentation and nearly shouted at me, "Jackson, what did he just say?" Fortunately, I was listening with one ear while looking with one eye. I calmly told him everything the other student had just said. Dr. Bradham gave me a smirk and told the other student to continue.

Later that day at lunch, Dr. Bradham and I were sitting in the students' and residents' chart room writing in our charts when suddenly he banged his hand down on the table and stared intently at me. I just about jumped out of my skin. As I said, he was a big man who had a habit of always pushing his lab coat up to his elbows, exposing his strong, hairy forearms. Startled, I looked at him bewildered. He hadn't shaved that day, and he had bushy chest hair creeping up over his top shirt button. "You know your dad never drank alcohol."

Not knowing where this was going, I hesitantly responded, "Yes, sir. I know that."

"He was a teetotaler all of his life?"

"Yes, sir. I'm pretty sure that's right."

"When I knew him, he was a resident, and he always brought his Pepsi to every social event so no one would ever think that he was drinking booze. Did you know that?"

"Yes, sir. I've heard about that."

"Damnedest thing I ever saw." Then he stopped and stared at me awhile. "How come you aren't scared of me like these other students?"

Now it was my turn to stare at him. I thought to myself, *Where did that come from, and what does it have to do with anything?* I smiled cautiously and replied, "I guess it's because you're just like my dad. You're intense, you're serious, and you demand excellence. I've been around that all of my life. I guess you'd say I'm accustomed."

He pondered that for a moment and then he asked, "Was Robert as serious a Christian as you?"

A little bit surprised, I asked, "Dr. Bradham, how do you know about my spiritual life?"

"I make it my business to know everything about the students on my service."

It was now my turn to be serious and intense. I guess I got that from my dad. "Dr. Bradham, my dad and I were on a spiritual growth curve before he died. We had numerous serious conversations about our relationship with the Lord the summer before he died. I watched how he related to his patients with a lovingkindness and a servant's heart that I believe only comes from the Lord. I'm still having a really hard time understanding why God took him."

He stood up, put his hand on my shoulder, and said, "Robert was a good man — a good doctor. You should be proud of him. Strive to be just like him." As he turned to leave, he said, "You know he always walked like he was walking through a freshly plowed field." Then he smiled at me and he was gone.

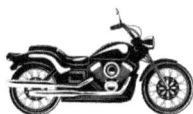

14

THE MARKSMAN

When I was a kid, Dad often went into the backyard with a Red Ryder BB gun and flipped a silver dollar up into the air. As it reached its apex, he shot it with a BB, practicing until he nailed it every time. When proficient with the silver dollar, he switched to a fifty-cent piece, and then subsequently a quarter and then, ultimately a dime, eventually shooting them all with precision.

My parents loved to entertain with outdoor cookouts, at which time Dad brought out his BB gun and entertained his guests with his BB gun marksmanship. He often allowed the other guests to try their hand at shooting the silver dollar, but without hours of practice, most could not even hit the silver dollar. Amazing his guests, Dad worked his way down from the silver dollar to shooting a dime out of the sky. His final act of showmanship was to throw a large washer up in the air, claiming he had shot through the middle of the washer when it reached its peak. Of course, the gathered crowd was incredulous. Therefore, he put black electrical tape over the hole in the middle of the washer and asked a guest to toss it up in the air for him; then he shot at it with the BB gun. When retrieved, sure enough a shiny copper BB lay embedded in the middle of the electrical tape, to everyone's delight. (He loved performing that feat, and he was really good at it.)

He was especially good at skeet shooting and bird hunting with a shotgun. Every year during the fall, his farming brothers conducted dove hunts, essentially large social events to which they invited all of their friends to gather around a large, recently harvested cornfield for the purpose of dove hunting. Beginning on Labor Day, these events occurred just about every Saturday in September and October. In the Lowcountry of South Carolina, these months were usually still scorching hot, so the host drove around in a pickup truck with coolers of ice-cold sodas in the back to slake the thirst of their guests.

About 1:00 on a particularly hot Thursday afternoon one September, I sat in Mr. Fuller's eighth grade literature class after lunch. The classroom was hot, the air was still and stuffy, and I was nodding off when my friend Freddie tapped me on the shoulder. I looked over my shoulder and spied my dad at the back door of the classroom, motioning for me to come there. My heart sank. The last time that happened, I was in the fourth grade in Mrs. Barnes's class. I was cutting fool with Freddie Spigner and Larry McCord when my dad just happened to be passing through, and here he was again at the very same classroom four years later! Only this time I wasn't messing around — that I knew of. I was just sleeping. *Oh, grabs!*

Wide awake now, I forced a smile and quick-stepped to the back of the class with all eyes following me, the very same eyes that saw me get taken to the little boys' room four years prior. I'm sure they were wondering, *What has he done now?* Well, so was I!

I got to the back door, and my dad whispered, "Go get your stuff. We're going dove hunting." I let out a huge sigh of relief, and my forced smile turned into a real smile.

I swaggered back to my seat, grabbed my books, and whispered to Freddie loud enough for everyone to hear, "Going dove hunting. See you later, chump."

Thursday was my dad's afternoon off from work. Dove and quail hunting were two of his passions in life. As previously mentioned, he was an excellent marksman, whether skeet shooting or bird hunting. Sadly, for me, I was blind as a bat and didn't know it until I applied for my driver's license at age sixteen. I dreaded the dove hunts because my dad and my uncles were all excellent shots, and I couldn't hit the broad side of a barn.

My dad would give me two boxes of shells, stick me in a prime spot on the side of a cornfield, and say, "Go get 'em, Cowboy." He would come back at the end of the afternoon, and I would be out of shells and have only two birds to show for it. It was totally embarrassing. He would just shake his head in disbelief. All afternoon, I would hear, "Robin, over your head, over your head!" I would look up and hear the unmistakable sound of doves flying overhead but would see nothing. I sometimes just threw my gun up and shot at the sound. How depressing! Then I would hear one of my uncles shout, "You've got to lead 'em, son; you've got to lead 'em, then follow through," as if my dad hadn't told me that a hundred times.

One particular day stands out in my mind. We were hunting a field prepared by my uncle Scott out near Paxville. We were all dispersed around the field. Dad had a two-way radio he used for hospital emergencies. He positioned himself in the middle of this large field and squatted in some cornstalks. Ten minutes later, the doves started flying furiously. I watched in fascination as Dad shot twelve times and bagged twelve birds. Other hunters whooped and hollered all around the cornfield at his demonstration of shooting expertise. They say that a good dove hunter will have a 50 percent shot success rate. Dad was 100 percent that day and had his limit in fifteen minutes. About that time, he received a call from the hospital and had to leave. He was gone for an hour and a half, during which time no birds flew at all. The rest of us just sat in the sweltering heat. There I sat — terribly bored, sweating, swatting gnats, and wondering why I subjected myself to such torture.

Ninety minutes later, Dad arrived back at the cornfield, resumed his position in the middle of the field, and asked one of my cousins if he could help him bag his limit. My cousin was no better shot than I was, so he replied, "Sure, Uncle Robert." I promise you on a whole case of 12-gauge shotgun shells, in ten minutes the birds started flying again, and in another fifteen minutes Dad had his limit with less than fifteen shots. Once again, grown men all around the field were exuberant at his shooting exhibition.

Then his radio crackled and he left for the hospital once again. He was gone for an hour or so and returned once more. While he was gone, only a few birds flew and only a few shots were fired. I continued to sit in boredom and did not see any of the birds that flew. When he returned this time, he walked over to me and asked, "You need help with getting your limit?"

I glumly jerked a broken corn stalk out of the ground, beat the root ball against the ground and replied, "I haven't even shot but twice all day. Have at it." He went to the same spot as before, knelt down in the cornstalks, and waited. True to form, in fifteen minutes the birds flew in like stealth bombers. He shot fourteen times and bagged twelve birds in about twenty minutes. His spectacular shooting had all of the hunters yelling in disbelief and admiration.

That was not the only time I saw him shoot in spectacular fashion.

One Saturday morning when I was sixteen years old, my dad woke me early and said, "Come on, boy. We're going quail hunting."

"But I'm still sleeping" was my response.

"You can sleep when you get to heaven."

I thought about that for a microsecond, then responded, "There ain't no sleeping in heaven. The lights are always on."

He was already fully dressed in brush pants and camo shirt and was walking briskly down the hall toward the kitchen. He responded over his receding shoulder, "Well, you can find out when you get there. Get dressed."

My dad was a doctor, an ex-Vietnam vet, a major in the Air National Guard, and no-nonsense. I got dressed quickly.

We arrived at my uncle Scott's farm to find several horses saddled up and two dogs in the back of his truck barking constantly. My uncle was intensely proud of his national field trial champion bird dogs. They were stout, muscular, and could run all day long. This November morning was cold and crisp with crystal blue skies. Not familiar at all with horses, I watched the older men tighten their cinches before climbing on. I pretended to know what I was doing as I fiddled with my horse's cinch. It became evident that I was clueless momentarily. When everyone saddled up, my saddle went sideways, dumping me hard on the ground. It knocked the breath out of me, but I was a football player, so I was accustomed to that. After the initial concern was over, we rode off, and I heard my uncle say, "Did you see how fast he fell off that horse?" Then I heard peals of laughter. I wasn't certain this was going to be a good day.

The two dogs took off running, scouting the edges of mature pines, occasionally stopping to sniff the air, and then off running again. Since we rode horses, we could cover a whole lot more territory and keep up with those dogs that were running machines. It wasn't long before Babe, the lead dog, pointed on the edge of the pines. Reb (short for Rebel) was soon locked in a point at a ninety-degree angle about fifteen yards away. We quickly dismounted, shouldered our shotguns, and quick-stepped behind the frozen-in-place bird dogs, both of whom trembled with excitement.

"Whoa, Babe. Easy, Reb," my uncle soothingly said as we approached — me in the middle and my dad and uncle on either side. Suddenly, with an explosion of whirring wings, about twelve quail leaped out of the broom straw and fled. My uncle Scott dropped two on the right. Dad dropped two on the left. My heart jumped into my throat. I never moved an inch. Paralyzed by the sudden noise and action, I never even pushed off the safety.

Dad shouted, "I got two."

Uncle Scott shouted, "I got two."

Then Dad, "Three by the biggest pine on the left, one by that large stump."

Scott shouted, "Two over there by that ditch. The rest are gone."

They were marking the birds that got away. I didn't see any of that. All I saw was a cloud of gun smoke and feathers flying as I stood rooted to the ground. The dogs came back up with big smiles on their faces and mouths full of quail. My dad just looked at me and shook his head.

In a minute, Babe was on two of the escapees. As we tiptoed up behind her, I was ready this time. Babe's head was low to the ground and tail straight up in the air, muscles twitching. The birds jumped up lightning fast. I fired my 20-gauge quickly before the bird was two feet off the ground and unfortunately only a foot over Babe's head. The bird was denuded and completely cleaned in an explosion of feathers. The hair on Babe's head stood straight up, but she never moved an inch. But not Uncle Scott. He screamed like a ten-year-old girl at her first horror movie. Babe was his prized, Blue Ribbon, national field trial champion bird dog, and I almost blew her brains out. He dropped to his knees and hugged the dog around the neck, looking at me in dismay. Both he and my dad began to berate me in the strongest terms, telling me how not to shoot a bird dog. I was right. This was not going to be a good day.

Both Uncle Scott and my dad were close to their limit in short order. I had my one naked bird plus two others. Reb pointed in a briar patch in mid-morning. Dad walked up behind him just as two quail tried to escape, but Dad, lightning fast, dropped them both before they got twenty yards away. Feathers floated slowly to the ground. Then surprisingly, a third bird shot straight up, flew in a confused circle, and turned right toward my dad. In self-defense, he thrust the butt of his 12-gauge at the bird, striking it in mid-air and turning it around. As it flew directly away from him, Dad shouldered his shotgun and nailed it, adding more feathers to those already floating to the ground. We all whooped and hollered. What a great day after all!

While in Manning on Christmas break in 1955, J.J. Britton, one of Robert's closest friends in high school, college, and later in medical school, discovered a duck pond in Elloree, South Carolina, that was loaded with ducks. He called Robert one evening before Christmas, "Hey, Robert, J.J. here. You wanna go duck hunting tomorrow morning?"

"Sure. Can I take John, my brother-in-law?"

"Yeah. Y'all be ready at 5:00 a.m. I'll pick you up. I'll have decoys. It'll take us forty minutes to get there."

"Where are we going?" Robert questioned.

"Can't tell you. It's my secret honey hole! But you'll love it. It's loaded with ducks."

"All right, we'll be ready," Robert responded with eager anticipation.

J.J. picked them up at 5:00 on the dot in his mother's car and drove them to Elloree, South Carolina. They parked on the side of a rural state road and backed up into some trees.

"OK, we'll walk from here," J.J. said.

"How far?" Robert inquired, staring into the cold black darkness of the predawn sky.

"About a half mile," J.J. replied, gathering his gun and decoys.

"Why can't we park closer?" John asked.

"You'll see," J.J. answered, already walking down the road with his decoy bag slung over his shoulder. They all walked a quarter mile down the state road, then turned right onto a dirt road leading through a freshly cut soybean field. Another quarter mile and they stood on the edge of a large pond three quarters surrounded by hardwoods. The pond seemed to go deeper into the woods like a swamp.

Taking charge, J.J. pointed his flashlight in the direction of the woods and said, "There's a dam about 150 yards down that way. I'll stand here on the shallow end. Y'all go down toward the dam; pick a good spot, and we'll wait until daylight. The ducks will start coming in right after daylight."

"All right, sounds like a good plan," replied Robert and John in unison as they set off in lockstep toward the barely visible dam. About twenty minutes later as the predawn darkness began to fade, John poked Robert and pointed at a sign on a tree forty yards away that clearly read, "POSTED — NO HUNTING."

John looked at his older brother-in-law and asked seriously, "You reckon he knows these people?"

"He must, or he wouldn't have brought us here."

John looked around a little uncertainly, then said, "Well, we're committed now. Here come the ducks." Sure enough, in twos and threes the ducks were coming in. In short order, it sounded like a small war on both ends of the pond. Shot gun blasts were followed by whoops and hollers.

"I got one."

"Whooee, John got a double!"

Suddenly, J.J. saw a long black sedan pull into the soybean field with headlights on. He hollered at John and Robert, but they just kept on shooting and hollering. J.J. stopped shooting and hunkered down behind some low-lying shrubs as the black sedan drove slowly by with two older men inside, looking all around with rather stern expressions. The shooting at the other end of the pond suddenly ceased amidst loud splashing. The black sedan slowly pulled out a few minutes later and disappeared down the state road.

After waiting about thirty minutes, J.J. gathered his decoys and eased back up the road to his mother's car. He slowly began to drive up and down country roads looking for his beleaguered friends. As he drove slowly along looking right and left, suddenly two drowned rats lurched out of the briars on the side of the road and dove into the back seat carrying firearms and dead ducks. Turns out they had to practically swim across the deep end of the pond to escape detection, carrying their ducks and firearms above their heads. They then shivered in the cold winter morning on the side of the road, waiting for their dubious benefactor to rescue them. Since John Land later became a state senator, J.J. never talked about this adventure that he shared with his good friend Robert Jackson until many years later when he heard Senator Land tell the story himself at a lunch meeting entertaining some of his legislative colleagues. Funny thing, of all the stories my dad ever told me, this wasn't one of them!

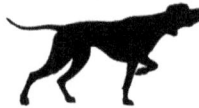

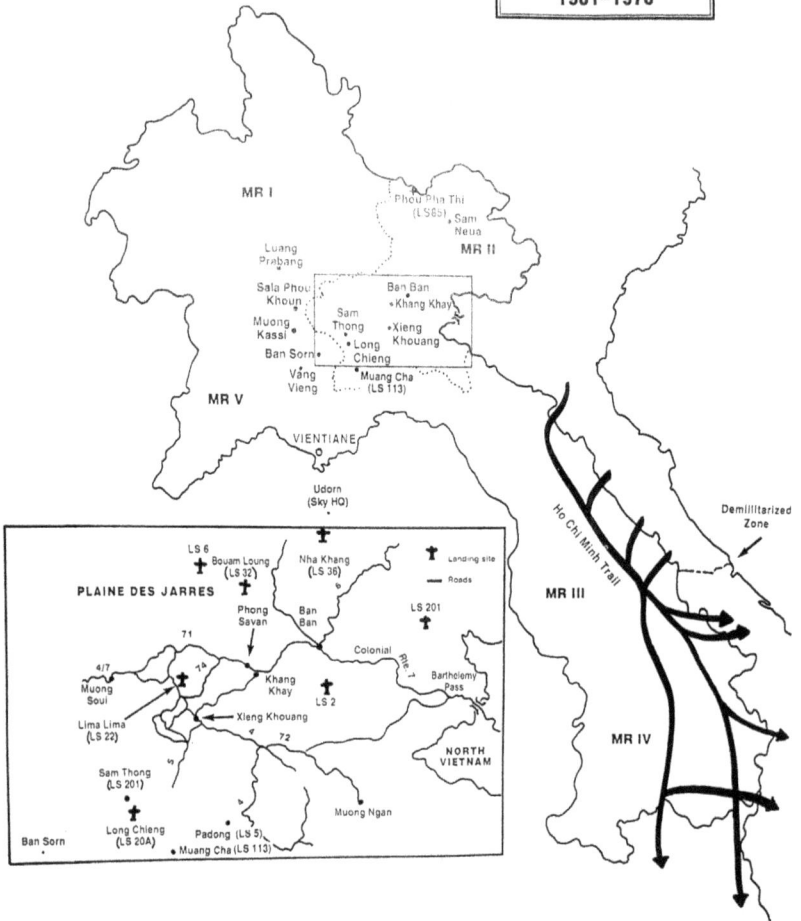

Laos: The Ground War
1961-1975

MR I

Phou Pha Thi
(LS 85), Sam
Neua

Luang
Prabang   MR II

Sala Phou   Ban Ban
Khoun   •Khang Khay
              Sam
Muong   Thong   •Xieng
Kassi   Khouang
            •Long
Ban Sorn•   Chieng

Vang   •Muang Cha
Vieng   └·····(LS 113)

MR V

VIENTIANE

Udorn   Demilitarized
(Sky HQ)   Zone

LS 6
    ✝ Bouam Loung   Nha Khang   ✝ Landing site
      (LS 32)   (LS 36)
PLAINE DES JARRES ✝   —— Roads

              Phong   Ban   LS 201
              Savan   Ban   ✝   MR III
    71
                         Colonial
    4/7   Bartholemy
Muong   Khang   Pass
Soui   Khay   ✝
Lima Lima   LS 2
(LS 22)   •Xieng Khouang
                    72   MR IV
                          NORTH
Sam Thong   VIETNAM
(LS 201)

    ✝   Muong Ngan

Ban Sorn Long Chieng Padong (LS 5)
          (LS 20A)   • Muang Cha (LS 113)

From Tragic Mountains: The Hmong, the Americans,
and the Secret Wars for Laos, 1942-1992

15

OFF TO WAR

With the winds of war blowing bitterly across the American landscape, Robert received notice that he, along with other young medical doctors, was about to be drafted into the military to serve American interests in the escalating conflict in Southeast Asia. He had a strong preference for serving in the Air Force, so he enlisted with them to guarantee his service in that branch of the military.

After basic training at Fort Maxwell in Alabama, he desired to be a part of the elite special forces, so he signed up to be a part of the Air Commandos, which required additional training in jungle and sea survival skills prior to his deployment to Southeast Asia. I recall him describing his experiences in jungle survival school. He and his fellow commandos were dropped into the jungle in Panama in groups of two with a .22 rifle and two shells only; then they navigated through the jungle to a prearranged location, which took about one week, while foraging for food and using a rudimentary map for navigation. He told me, "We were about to starve on the last day when we spied a large iguana, shot him with the .22 rifle, and cooked him over an open fire. It was the best meat I have ever eaten after four days of eating fruit and berries." They arrived at their rendezvous point none the worse for wear and survived the jungle.

The Air Commandos also attended a jump school where they mastered jumping from "perfectly good airplanes." Dad took me to the jump school, where, as an eleven-year-old boy, I watched with utter fascination as his classmates jumped from towers, learned to land without injuring themselves, and learned to pack their parachutes.

Dad's basic and special forces training required about six months' time, during which my sister, Anne, and I lived with my Grandmother and Grandfather Land in Manning so we could finish our respective years in grade school. During that time, I became very close to Lillie Mae, my grandmother's housekeeper and cook. She was a short, overweight black woman who could always make me laugh with her joviality; plus, she and I talked about life in general every day after school, including my dad's training for the war. On Saturday mornings when I wasn't in school, she would hike up her skirt, roll down her knee-high stocking, remove a few dollar bills and some coins, and then dispatch me down to Dan's Shell Station to purchase for her a quarter's worth of snuff. I had no idea what snuff was, but the men loitering at Dan's thought it quite humorous that the doctor's boy bought snuff. Years later, I realized they may have thought I was purchasing it for my very aristocratic grandmother, which then made me belly laugh.

After Dad returned from his military service, Lillie Mae's twenty-four-year-old son, Vesti Driggers, was deployed in July of 1968 to South Vietnam as an Army infantryman. I happened to be at my grandmother's home one autumn day in 1968 when two stern men in uniform knocked on my grandmother's front door and asked for Lillie Mae. Bewildered, I informed her of our guests, and with trembling lips and a terrified visage she walked ever so slowly to the front door. When she saw their uniforms, she shrieked and began to wail, "Lord God Almighty, no, no, nooo!" They handed her a telegram as she slumped to the floor. They spoke a few words that neither she nor I heard over her wailing. I was speechless and paralyzed. Thankfully, someone must have notified Grandma, because shortly she arrived and took charge. Lillie Mae's son drowned on November 29, 1968, while crossing a river on a routine patrol in Thua Thien Province, South Vietnam.

My recollection is that Grandmother Land attended the wake a few days later with one other friend and commented to me with a note of disappointment that they were the only Caucasians in attendance at the memorial service for a young black soldier who died in the war while serving our country. This highly emotional event and the image of the two men in uniform standing at my grandmother's front door could have just as easily played out in the life of our family as it did in many other families across our state and nation. Pondering my dad's service and Vesti's sacrifice, I would never forget the potential consequences of military service. Indeed, the tears flowed just writing this. I didn't know Vesti, but I knew Lillie Mae and I shared her grief. At thirteen years old, it left a long-lasting impression on my life.

Before long, Dad's training concluded, the whole family returned to Manning, and he headed to Southeast Asia for six months of a life-changing high adventure. The family settled in for six months of dread, knowing he was in the danger zone. Already the nightly newscasts reported the tales of carnage in South Vietnam, portraying graphic images of dead or wounded American soldiers returning from there. The entire extended Jackson family worried and fretted over their youngest sibling-turned-soldier, but none as much as Abbot — who continued to care for four small children all alone and worried every day about her husband's safety, especially since he was on special assignment in a location that he could not disclose. Her angst was mitigated somewhat by the day-to-day routine of caring for the children, but a heavy pall lay over the entire household due to the uncertainty of the times and lack of information regarding his status.

It was years later before Abbot actually knew Robert's exact location in Southeast Asia, because his location was classified. His letters home arrived erratically, usually in collections of six to ten at a time. All names and locations were redacted for years until the military permitted Robert to fill in the blanks, allowing Abbot to understand where he was and with whom he was affiliated.

After arriving in Southeast Asia, Robert was assigned to serve in Laos as part of America's secret war against Communism by supporting the Hmong, a people who "disliked the Vietnamese and desired to be free." The 1954 Geneva Conference divided Vietnam into North and South — and declared Laos, formerly under French control for over fifty years, to be an independent state under the rule of the Royal Lao Government. At the same time, the pro-Communist Pathet Lao established their presence in two northern Laotian provinces. Civil war broke out, with the Soviet Union and Pathet Lao supporting one faction. Because the political situation destabilized and because the Soviet Union stepped in, President Eisenhower and his Secretary of State, John Dulles, worried that Laos could fall to Communism, resulting in a "domino effect" leading to the fall of Thailand and the rest of Southeast Asia. They had been sending economic and military aid via air support, but eventually decided to accept a CIA suggestion to step up United States involvement by coming alongside Hmong tribesmen in their efforts against the Communists rather than sending American troops. The Geneva Conference reaffirmed Laos' neutral status in July 1962. In accordance with this agreement, the United States withdrew its military support of the Hmong; however, it soon became obvious that the North Vietnamese did not pull their 7,000 troops from Laos. More than that, they continued to fight for control over the people of Laos, and they continued to use the Ho Chi Minh trail through Laos and Cambodia to transport critical military supplies to the Viet Cong in South Vietnam.

After being recruited by the CIA for their covert operation in Laos, Robert reported to the United States Embassy in Vientiane, Laos, where he had to divest himself of any affiliation with the American military since the Americans had no official presence in Laos. There he turned in his Air Force uniform and all identification. Thereafter, he was referred to in military reports as "Number One." If captured or killed, he would most likely be identified as a volunteer with USAID, which was headquartered in Sam Thong. As mentioned previously, it appeared as if he worked under

the auspices of USAID, basically a humanitarian organization helping the
Laotian people and cooperating with Air America. William Leary summa-
rizes Air America's activities with:

> Air America was a vital component in the [CIA's] opera-
> tions in Laos. By the summer of 1970, the airline had some two
> dozen twin-engine transports, another two dozen short-take-
> off-and-landing (STOL) aircraft, and some thirty helicopters
> dedicated to operations in Laos. There were more than 300 pilots,
> copilots, flight mechanics, and air-freight specialists flying out
> of Laos and Thailand. During 1970, Air America airdropped or
> landed 46 million pounds of foodstuffs — mainly rice — in Laos.
> Helicopter flight time reached more than 4,000 hours a month in
> the same year. Air America crews transported tens of thousands
> of troops and refugees, flew emergency medevac missions and
> rescued downed airmen throughout Laos, inserted and extracted
> road-watch teams, flew nighttime airdrop missions over the Ho Chi
> Minh Trail, monitored sensors along infiltration routes, conducted
> a highly successful photo-reconnaissance program, and engaged
> in numerous clandestine missions using night-vision glasses and
> state-of-the-art electronic equipment. Without Air America's
> presence, the CIA's effort in Laos could not have been sustained.

Robert was assigned to the San Sook Hospital located in northern Laos
at Sam Thong, where he would be the flight surgeon for American air crews
shot down over North Vietnam who were instructed to escape to Laotian
territory where friendly forces could rescue them. Additionally, he cared
for the friendly forces that used the airfield where the medical facility was
located. The hospital site included a 2,000-foot dirt airstrip for bringing
in supplies and wounded soldiers; a steady stream of both arrived just
about every day. Constructed by the USAID program in 1964, the 100-bed

hospital was initially operated by two Filipino doctors, but their service to the local Meo and Lao people was unacceptable. They were asked to leave, but damage had already been done. The locals were very reluctant to go to the hospital due to the precedence of poor care set by these doctors. Enter Captain Jackson and a French-trained Laotian surgeon named Dr. Khammoung (Dr. K.).

Colonel Charles E. Ramsey recalled the first time he met Captain Jackson:

> He came into the operations building in Udorn, Thailand, where I was the commander of the 606 Detachment of the Air Commandos. He gave a sharp salute and said, "I'm Robert Jackson, the new flight surgeon sent over to join the detachment."
>
> The way he said it, I thought to myself, *My God, who is this eager beaver? I guess he hasn't been over here long enough to know what the hell it's all about.* He was a lot of energy and looking for something to do.
>
> The flight surgeon before Bob [Robert] had stuck close to the detachment and had been satisfied with the local sick calls and such. Not Bob [Robert]. The first thing he wanted to know was, "When can I go up-country?"
>
> In case you don't know where "up-country" is, I'm not going to tell you now [this was classified information at the time], but I will say that it's the kind of hellhole that no one in civilization liked to live in, and most self-respecting, money-making doctors would not be caught dead in. Well, Bob [Robert] isn't that sort. I never really knew whether he liked it there because he was helping someone else or he was learning something new. I know part of it was helping someone else, but he used to tell me that he learned more in a month, and saw more unusual cases, than most doctors did in a lifetime in the States. He said it like he was lucky.

After being stationed in Sam Thong, Dad wrote in a journal regarding his daily activities, including the following entries:

7/19/66 — North Country — Another day is ending. I processed through the embassy office today. I had to get rid of all Air Force identification. At 7:00 a.m., I take off for the hospital. ... This hospital is on the original site that Tom Dooley started. It is located 120 miles behind enemy lines, therefore, the necessity of air travel. No roads are available across the mountains. It is still a very secure place because the geography of the area protects it from all sides.

7/20/66 — Sam Thong, Laos — Well, I finally made it here. I left Vientiane at 7:30 a.m., and we flew over the mountains to Sam Thong where the hospital is located. It is situated in a valley with a 2,000-foot runway. The surrounding area looks exactly like the Blue Ridge Mountains. It is ten-to-twenty degrees cooler here than in Udorn. Of course, there is red clay mud everywhere because of the daily rains.

The hospital is of wooden construction and is spread out in four different directions. Each portion of the hospital is one big room with wooden cots lining the walls, each cot covered by a straw mat. There are approximately 120 beds here. I made rounds with Dr. Khammoung, a Laotian doctor, who is a partially trained surgeon. ... The patients are either Lao or Meo tribesmen. As you know, the Lao and Meo are at war against the Communist-backed Pathet Lao. Nearly all of the medically sick people had malaria, the first cases I had ever seen. All had very enlarged spleens.

LATER: I had to stop writing as a helicopter just landed and off-loaded a sick man. He has bronchial pneumonia and acute malaria, my first solo case. A site near here is under attack so I can expect wounded any time now. Helicopters will bring them into the hospital. There is one operating room with a single portable overhead light. The OR nurse is a Filipino who speaks broken English.

In a report that Captain Jackson submitted to Strategic Air Command at a later date: "Each ward in the hospital has running water and a lavatory. The water supply is obtained from a mountain stream near the hospital. (The water traveled down a bamboo pipe and was then filtered through gauze to remove sand particles.) All water for drinking has to be boiled and filtered. Electricity is supplied by a diesel-powered generator.

"The sterilizer is an army-type run by butane gas. There are minimal lab facilities. Each patient's family moves into the hospital with the patient and provides food and nursing care. There are several young Laotian girls who have been taught to dispense medicines. Also, two Lao Army medics are there who give shots, change dressings, etc. The Laotian surgeon is competent and friendly. I am glad he is here.

More journal entries in his own words:

7/23/66 — The water for the shower is ice cold. I do not know what I will do when winter comes. There is also no heater. The drinking water has to be filtered and boiled before drinking.

The hospital care is for the majority of the people of this country and by far the larger number of casualties. I wear only a pair of jungle fatigues and a T-shirt up here. In the OR, our boots are left on covered with the mud. I do put on a scrub shirt, cap, and sterile gloves. I am sure that Dr. Schweitzer in Africa or Dr. Seagrave, the Burma surgeon, never had it this good. We even did a blood transfusion yesterday.

This has been the busiest day so far. We admitted seven soldiers today. Three had acute malaria; the others had lower extremity injuries. One had to have a BK [below knee] amputation. Another with a fracture of the femur had debridement and a Steinman pin inserted in the distal tibia for traction. The other had a large through-and-through wound in the thigh, which I just debrided thoroughly and left open because it had some degree of infection. I performed the surgery under spinal anesthesia. I am learning fast and gaining valuable experience.

You would be amazed at the activity in this place. There is an airplane landing here every five-to-ten minutes all day. They haul rice, refugees, wounded, etc. There is a continuous movement of planes. These pilots deserve a lot of credit. They are civilians working for Air America or Continental Air Transport. All flights are over enemy territory, and many of the planes get shot at and occasionally one goes down. When I fly up here to visit our medics at the various outposts, it will count as a combat mission. [Robert ultimately accumulated over ninety combat missions flying over hostile enemy territory.]

7/24/66 — The work here gets more interesting each day. Today I did a laparotomy for an ectopic pregnancy with Dr. K's assistance. Also, a soldier came in with three fingers on each hand shattered by a detonator cap. Dr. K. operated on one hand and I on the other. The tips were amputated, then closed. Early this morning, we drained a psoas muscle abscess. Also, I corrected a child's deformed fifth finger.

The patients in the hospital sleep on a wooden bed like a table about two feet off the floor. The mattresses are thin straw mats covered by a blanket. There is no linen or pillow. The blankets are washed between patients. The patient's family comes to the hospital and stays there until he is discharged. Large French-type loaves of bread are flown in each day from Vientiane, and the loaves are distributed to the patients. The hospital cooks rice for all of the patients. The family of the patients have no plates, so they put fruit, rice, etc., on large green leaves and use the leaves to eat off.

When patients are brought by aircraft to the hospital, the airplanes taxi up to the front door, and the medics push a stretcher to the plane and offload the patient. I can look directly out the operating room window and see the planes bringing the wounded in. The OR floor is covered with a linoleum rug, which has a large piece missing right under the head of the operating room table, through which I can see pigs and chickens running under the OR. Mud now fills the cracks in the floor.

7/27/66 — Whenever a local person who has worked here at Sam Thong for any length of time has to leave, the native villagers have a ceremony in his honor, and they call it a *basi* (pronounced "baahsi"). They put fruit and flowers on the floor, and everyone sits around in a circle on the floor and eats fruit, pork, bread, or whatever they serve. They also have a local bootleg whiskey called *Lai Lai*, which is as potent as gasoline. If you stick a match to it, it will burn. Anyway, the honored guest is required to drink this explosive mixture. Another custom is to tie strands of white string around your wrist for good luck. The more strings they tie on you, the better they like you. You must wear these strings for at least three days. They held a *basi* last night at the Operational Quonset Hut for Sam Adams, who had been here for a year. They offered me a drink of *Lai Lai,* and I faked sipping on it and poured it out. The fumes were like fire. The bread, cookies, and fruit I ate without any trouble. Maybe they'll give me a *basi* before I leave, but if I were made to drink the *Lai Lai,* I would surely die.

8/3/66 — It is amazing how many Air Force and Army people are up here engaged in behind-the-lines counterinsurgency work. All are in constant danger of attack or capture. I hope that the good Lord will continue to watch over us all.

US Army Captain John Reid, one of Robert's housemates at Sam Thong, shared this account of meeting the new doctor:

One day, I came into the village and heard that a new Air Force doctor had just arrived and was at the hospital. I went down to greet him but, before I could say anything, he had me lying down on a native-style bamboo bed with a needle in my arm. He then told me that he had a local soldier who had been shot through the back and stomach several days earlier. I asked how he knew my blood type would match the soldiers. He said that any kind would do when the soldier had none otherwise. Robert had already transfused more than a normal amount from his arm directly into the unconscious soldier. After using my blood, the patient still needed more. Robert claimed that he could still barely hear a pulse. He persuaded the other Americans present to donate blood, and the young soldier began to improve. The next day, Robert operated and found the soldier had been shot through the liver. His operation was successful, and the soldier was up walking around the hospital in a couple of days. This soldier eventually became a valuable assistant at the hospital until he was returned to his Army unit.

[Captain Reid and Captain Jackson were able to maintain their close friendship after their service in SEA when Captain Reid became a professor at Wofford College in Spartanburg, South Carolina. He invited Dr. Jackson on several occasions to Wofford to speak to his students.]

To address an interesting issue, here is a sentence from one letter:

8/9/66 — One of my patients died today after eating a handful of opium.

I refer to the book *Tragic Mountains* to describe what opium meant to the Laotian people and why Dad would mention this in his letters:

Life in the beautiful mountain country of Laos was harsh. It was not easy to earn a living from the steep mountainside fields. Many families tended patches of opium poppies, which grew best at elevations of over 3,000 feet. The harvest of opium was often their only cash crop, which was then used to purchase salt, pots, Chinese needles, and silk cloth.

Traditionally, Hmong used opium as a natural medication, particularly for diarrhea, stomach disorders, fevers, and pain. Hmong either grew their own opium or traded for it. Elderly Hmong sometimes smoked opium to induce sleep or to ease the aches and pains of age. While, as a rule, Hmong were not drug abusers, addiction did occur, but it was frowned upon. An opium addict was a burden to his family, his village, and his clan.

The dry season was the time to harvest the opium pods. Women and children, using small, curved knives, made two or three slits on each hardened poppy pod. White sap oozed from the cuts. Exposed to air, the strong-smelling sap turned dark. This was raw opium. Harvesters, often with their noses and mouths covered to protect themselves from the strong odor of the sap, moved slowly through hillside poppy fields, laboriously scraping small bubbles of sap from pods into leaves. Each pod produced only a minuscule amount of sap. A family poppy field could not provide much income. It is surprising how much effort was required to harvest a small field of poppy, which produced, if the weather was just right, one to two kilograms of opium.

While Hmong had traditionally grown opium poppies and had used opium as a medicine, they had never converted opium into heroin nor marketed it to the world. During colonial times, the French opium monopoly purchased the opium, which was channeled into the medicinal market as morphine. The French government however, decided to give up its opium monopoly, so Chinese traders had access to the entire opium production of Laos.

Dad also mentioned the following to contrast the traditional medical care the mountain people commonly received to the modern care that he and Dr. K. provided at the San Sook Hospital:

8/9/66 — A little girl was brought in today with a rectal problem/infection. The local witch doctor had pushed some leaves into the rectum to stop diarrhea.

His letters continue:

8/21/66 — This morning, Dr. K. and I removed a varicocele in an adult male. Around noon, a soldier was brought in who had terrible wounds of both hands, face, and left leg as the result of a land-mine explosion. He lost all fingers on the right hand except the thumb, and on his left hand he lost the thumb plus the index and middle finger. He was also blinded in the right eye. It took two and a half hours of surgery to repair all of his injuries.

8/29/66 — Today has been one that you read about in fiction books. After leisurely rounds, we explored a female patient and discovered a hepatic cyst, which we drained. Before we finished with her, two helicopter loads of soldiers arrived. Three had minor wounds, but the other was shot through the liver. He was in shock, no blood pressure, and very near death. We started an IV and then had to round up blood donors. A man came in with him and had the same type of blood but refused to donate. This made me mad, so I gave a pint for him and sent my medic over to

Site 21-A to get some blood over there. After two units of blood, his pressure was up enough to start the operation. I first explored his abdomen, and everything was OK. After closing the abdomen, I enlarged the wound of entrance and found a large tear in the liver and diaphragm plus two broken ribs. I cut away a portion of rib for better exposure; then I packed the liver with gel foam and sutured the liver capsule over the gel foam. Next, I repaired the torn diaphragm and sutured the wound. It was exciting surgery, and I enjoyed every minute of it.

8/30/66 — Today at the hospital, we saw about forty-nine outpatients plus debrided both legs of a burn patient. This afternoon, Dr. K. and I did a strangulated hernia with gangrene of the small bowel, which necessitated a resection and anastomosis. I did this one today. I have really progressed in the six weeks I have been up here, from never having done any major surgery up to today when I did the intestinal resection. That's a big jump in only six weeks.

Late yesterday, a man came in with a large cut on the forehead, which was three days old. He had grass stuck in the wound. Another lady came in with a severe wound of her leg, which she had filled with cow dung — of all things. A favorite treatment of these people is to tie grass or weeds around their waist or neck when they are sick.

8/31/66 — I have a soldier in traction for a fractured femur. It was necessary to put a little weight on his leg off to one side to align the broken ends properly. The weight was placed in a sack and tied to the leg and hung over the side of the bed. When I made rounds today, the leg was grotesquely crooked, and I couldn't understand why until I checked the bag with the small weight in it. Well, the patient had chosen the bag to store his goodies in, which included a quart of water, a piece of bread, and some rice. Such is life at our hospital!

One of our helicopters was fired on today, but only one bullet hit the chopper. You never know when you'll be shot at up here.

9/2/66 — About 3:00 p.m. today, the patients and the wounded really started coming in. We admitted several people with acute malaria, all of which had very big spleens. Five soldiers also came in — two with bullet wounds of the thigh, no fractures; another one with a compound fracture of the radius; and one with a shrapnel wound of the abdomen with perforation of the ileum. The other soldier had typhoid fever and peritonitis due to two perforations in his ileum. Dr. K. did the first perforation and I did the second. It has been a real busy day — the kind I like.

[Because of the desperate need for blood transfusions at the Sam Thong hospital,] I talked to Colonel Ramsey about periodically coming to Udorn and drawing blood from his troops to supply our blood bank up here. He is in agreement, so I guess I will be flying down to Udorn one day to draw blood. I would put it on ice and fly right back up here with it.

9/6/66 — On Friday of this week, Bob (Kosha) and I are to fly to Udorn and draw twenty pints of blood for our hospital. I sent Colonel Ramsey a note today to have the donors assembled at his place at 1:00 p.m. Friday. I hope it all works out because we sure need the blood.

My moustache is quite long now. When I was in Udorn Sunday picking up items for the hospital, everyone stared at me like I was a nut. Everyone there was clean-shaven and dressed in standard military attire with clean, starched and pressed uniforms. There I was with my old commando hat on, my moustache, my hunting knife on my side plus rugged outdoor clothing. No one doubted me when I told them I worked up North. We never say "Laos," just "up North." As you know, at Sam Thong I am designated "Number One" — not captain or doctor.

9/7/66 — A "Jolly Green Giant" rescue chopper came into the hospital at 5:30 p.m. with two seriously injured on board. One young soldier was shot in the abdomen and through the pelvis, plus had a severe laceration and fracture of his foot. The other had a compound fracture of his right leg, plus multiple shrapnel wounds. I explored the first man and found a lacerated gall bladder and omental hematoma. Two of his toes had to be amputated. The other man was cleaned up, and his wounds debrided and his fractured leg splinted. Before we could finish with these two, seven more wounded came in. All had multiple shrapnel wounds, but none required extensive surgery. All in all, we admitted fifteen soldiers today. There is only one vacant bed left in the hospital now. The injured yesterday and today resulted from an offensive started up north of here. It has been dry for five days, and I knew this increased activity would result in more casualties.

9/9/66 — Bob (Kosha) and I flew down to Udorn today and drew twenty-two pints of blood for the hospital. It is comforting to have a reservoir of blood. When we returned around 5:00 p.m., there were six wounded in the OR, and poor Dr. K. was operating on another one all alone.

9/10/66 — I saw my first case of leprosy today. The patient had involvement of the nerves and skin of his right arm with anesthesia (numbness) and deformity of the hand.

9/18/66 — We had an attack only twelve miles from here yesterday.

9/19/66 — Around noon today, I walked down to the marketplace and got a haircut. The barbershop was just a straw roof with poles around the sides — one straight chair, a mirror, and hand-operated clippers. I was a real curiosity, as about twenty-five people crowded around to see me, the American soldier, getting a haircut. After he finished with his clippers, he put soap around my ears, reached into his pocket, and pulled out a big pocketknife and used that to shave me. He did not just shave a little around the ears but shaved halfway up the side of my scalp. I am really skint, but feel better with my hair shorter.

9/21/66 — Today has been belly wound day. We have had two laparotomies to repair intestinal injuries. Dr. K. did the first. I just finished the second. In between the two laps, we had several other injured soldiers with various shrapnel wounds, plus one with a compound fracture of the left forearm. It is really a job to take care of the old patients, plus do all the necessary surgery. We could use another medical doctor just to look out after the medical patients and general duties. Since it has stopped raining, there is a continuous flow of patients to the hospital. We are again out of beds.

9/23/66 — About 8:00 p.m. tonight, a bomb was dropped very close to here. All of the buildings here were shaken by the blast. Of course, all of us were startled but fortunately no more have been heard. The war is rather close to us now, but I do not feel alarmed as yet.

9/24/66 — Later today, I was summoned to the village to see a woman who had just had a baby and was bleeding. When I arrived, she was sitting on a little stool with hot coals underneath. After much coaxing, she consented to lie down. Her blood pressure was 40/0. I gave her a unit of Dextran, and her blood pressure came up OK. The bleeding stopped after a Pitocin injection, and when I left, she was doing fairly well. In the morning, I will check on her again.

Colonel Ramsey also reported:

I often traveled up to see Bob (Robert) when I could because he wouldn't leave his patients to come down to at least mild civilization to see me unless I sent for him or unless something unusual was going on. When I was at Sam Thong, he always took me on rounds of the "hospital" with him, and I never got over the way all the patients would smile and hold out their hands to him as we went through the bare rooms with the bare wooden beds. I remember once when we walked out of the front door of the "hospital," there was a woman there who had her dead son wrapped in a cloth and lying on the floor. She was taking him home. When she saw Bob, she came over and grabbed his hands and kissed them with tears in her eyes, and said something that neither of us could understand. The boy was only twelve years old and had been shot by the Pathet Lao. She was thanking Bob for what he had done and had tried to do, not blaming him for not saving the only child she had.

More letters:

9/25/66 — I went back to check on the postpartum bleeder early this morning, and she is doing quite well. It is an improvement in relations between Americans and the natives when they send for the American doctor to treat them. I believe the villagers here have accepted me, as they all seem very happy to see me, and they no longer hesitate to come see me at the hospital for treatment. (This is in sharp contrast to the fearfulness they exhibited previously when the Filipino doctors were at San Sook Hospital.)

Five wounded came in today — three with multiple shrapnel wounds from a land-mine explosion, and one a woman with a five-year-old daughter; both had been shot by the VC [Viet Cong]. The woman had a large hole in her thigh. The child was shot through the forearm with both bones fractured. They all should do OK. Earlier today, we removed an eyeball from a woman who had lost her sight from a land-mine injury. The eye was very scarred and painful. A little child with contractures in two fingers had them released in the OR. *All in all, it was a very peaceful Sunday.* [The italics are mine as I thought it rather ironic for him to call this a "peaceful" day.]

Captain Reid, one of Robert's bunk mates, in a letter to Abbot, stated:

The most professional part of Robert's work at Sam Thong was the way that he handled the many casualties. Helicopters loaded with battle casualties arrived at the hospital almost daily. Robert assisted in unloading the casualties, then triaged those who needed to be treated immediately and continued to work as long as required until all that could be done for them was completed. His genuine concern for them was infectious and permeated the entire work force. This, in turn, changed the attitude of many of the locals about coming to Sam Thong hospital for medical treatment. The Laotians were accustomed to being treated by witch-doctor types from their own villages and hesitated to come to Sam Thong.

I feel certain that the official reason for Robert's assignment to Sam Thong was for the emergency treatment of the rescued pilots. However, the United States government's total effort in Laos was immeasurably helped by his work with and for the local mountain people.

Captain Reid's assessment was right on target. As documented by an after-action assessment submitted by Captain Jackson to First Air Commando Wing military commanders at a later date, his statement began:

Sir, this is top secret ... Medical civic action such as the program presently operating in South Vietnam under the auspices of the USAID program will greatly improve the general level of health and preventive medicine of the Laotian people. If a well-organized and directed unit of US trained medical personnel could be deployed to previously selected sites, a major barrier to the Communist advance in Laos would be achieved.

Medical civic action is an integral part of any effective counterinsurgency operation. The goodwill produced as a result of competent medical care would far offset the cost involved and certainly be more effective than arms and ammunition in obtaining the Laotian people's interest and support in the objectives of the US in Southeast Asia.

More statements from letters:

9/26/66 — We have six patients recovering from intestinal wounds, and all are doing well. I am really pleased that our belly wounds do well. When abdominal cases such as perforations and resections do well, this indicates good surgical techniques. Dr. K. has really taught me a wealth of surgery since I came here. I hope I can use some of this new knowledge later in my practice.

[Robert commented in a separate diary entry that the military doctor who preceded him at Sam Thong had left a multitude of patients with infected wounds. Therefore, it was all the more remarkable that under Robert's tenure there were no wound infections, despite many old and contaminated wounds upon the patients' arrivals.]

9/27/66 — All the post-op patients are progressing well. Since I arrived in July, there has not been a single abdominal wound infection in any of the laparotomy patients. This is quite remarkable in view of the surroundings here. We try to be as sterile as possible during all of the surgical procedures. All dressings are changed each day and the wounds closely inspected.

10/5/66 — Another exciting day! At 9:30 a.m. while making rounds, Pop [Pop Buell — USAID director] called me and told me to get ready to go up North to Site 36 right away. Well, 36 is pretty close to the North Vietnam border and in the middle of Communist country. I packed my emergency pack, including my flares, pistol, and survival radio. Site 36 is about sixty miles from here ... On arrival at 36, the first impression is shocking, because there are bomb craters all around the site from previous attacks. Outposts and trenches completely surround the area. Soldiers abound. When we landed, I was told that an F-4C jet plane with two crewmen aboard was shot down. A "Jolly Green Giant" rescue chopper went to pick them up and was driven away by ground fire. I later counted eight bullet holes in the chopper. One of the chopper crew was wounded, but not seriously. The rescue choppers are armor-plated around the pilots. If it were not so, maybe both pilots would be dead, and the chopper lost. Anyway, a second rescue attempt was made, and one of the pilots was picked up. He had a compound fracture of his left ankle and possible compression fractures of his back. He was brought to Site 36. I checked him over and placed him aboard a C-123 and flew with him to Udorn. I turned him over to the flight surgeon there. I really looked like an outdoor trooper with my jungle hat, knife, boots, and short-sleeved scrub shirt, plus carrying my emergency pack on my back.

The second pilot could not be reached. He was talking on the radio for a while; then he said he had been hit by ground fire and was passing out. That was his last communication.

10/12/66 — This afternoon I flew by helicopter to Site 108 to check on four wounded soldiers ... While I was there, Terry Collins, who worked for USAID, asked me to visit a few villages around there because of poor living conditions and generally poor health of the villagers. We first went to a small village accessible only by helicopter. It was located by a small river way up in the mountains. All of the houses were on stilts and made of bamboo. The village scene resembled a picture you would see in a *National Geographic* magazine. There were half-naked women with children tied on their backs. The entire population greeted us on our arrival. The village chief invited us into his house. I took off my shoes and went in. The people began to crowd into the little house until the bamboo floor began to sag and creak. Everyone had some kind of medical complaint. All of the children had malaria or worms. Several adults with tuberculosis were examined. I did not go prepared to treat a wealth of patients, so my medicines were soon out.

Next, we went to Site 57, which is adjacent to the enemy lines. From there we walked about a mile through the jungle to another village, which had only eleven shacks. We had to cross a bridge over the river. The bridge was made from logs — very shaky. The children and the adults all needed vitamins, deworming, and malaria medicine. These visits today have made me realize how much good could be accomplished by periodic visits to these areas. The enemy are all around these places. They do not bother with much daytime activity. The helicopter I was in today was fired at by ground fire just after I was let off at Site 57.

10/13/66 — The fighting has died down, as the soldiers on both sides are busy harvesting rice. When this is done in about two weeks, business should again pick up.

10/17/66 — I had hoped to be able to visit some of the nearby villages and treat the sick there, but Dr. Weldon says that the ambassador does not want me out in the countryside. Being military, I am not supposed to be here anyway. I guess that is one reason they took my name away and gave me a number.

10/28/66 — After working with these people who are so happy with the barest of essentials, it is saddening to think of the waste and greed of America. I am happy to have been able to contribute a small part to making their existence perhaps a little better and healthier.

11/13/66 — The big medical ward is completely filled, especially so with all the kinfolks sleeping in with the sick ones. One older lady is lying by her husband, and the two of them are both smoking opium. The opium is cooked over a small candle, and then placed in a big pipe and deep inhalations taken. Opium is a big business in this country.

11/15/66 — I spent several hours at Site 192. Again, I saw nearly 200 people, mostly with malaria. I dewormed nearly 100 children.

11/20/66 — I just cannot believe that everything is progressing so rapidly. The days up here are just flying by. I got scared last week, fearing that something was going to happen to me, especially when I was at Site 192. Oftentimes, I dream of the VC attacking and I awaken in a cold sweat.

In Captain John Reid's correspondence with Abbot:

I actually knew Robert only a few months in Laos. I saw him mostly in the evenings when I stopped at Sam Thong. He was such a delight to be around. I stayed in his little room next to the hospital and we frequently played darts at night. It was frustrating to me, but I could never beat him at darts.

Robert was certainly an inspiration to me. I wish I could have known him longer than those brief few months because I think all who were around him became better people. Because of his natural leadership skills, I felt that eventually Robert would become one of our political leaders. I never suspected him of being a politician, but because of his enormous capabilities he would be a natural. I expected one day to see him as governor.

An article in an Air Force publication in March 1967 described his war service as follows: "We know too well that the only way to stop the insidious advances of Communism is to win the hearts of the people — and medicine is more effective than bullets. Without a gun, Dr. Jackson fought a war — a war to win the people."

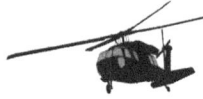

16

CELEBRITY STATUS

The following excerpt from *Tragic Mountains* illustrates the vital importance of the quality medical/surgical care provided at the San Sook Hospital at Sam Thong and the blood bank program initiated by Captain Jackson:

At dawn the next morning, (Hmong pilot) Vang Chou, as usual, discussed with the AOC commander Hmong reports of enemy movements and helped chart schedules for the day's Raven flights. (Raven flights were airborne forward air controllers, who could spot enemy installations and coordinate air strikes.) With Sam Deichalman in the left seat and Chou in the right, they flew into the greyness of the early morning for a long and dangerous day searching for the enemy. By noon, Sam and Chou had successfully marked two strikes and refueled at Alternate for the afternoon flight. As the afternoon wore on, Chou flew the plane from the right seat. Sam seemed exhausted. He pushed his seat back to relax and rest his eyes. Chou watched the weather and the time, ... As 3:00 approached, he headed toward heavily defended Ban Ban on Route 7.

Over the rendezvous site, Chou flew slowly at about 500 feet, looking for trucks. They were there just as he had predicted. Five of them. ... While keeping the five trucks in sight, he looked for more targets and noticed two bunkers dug into two facing hillsides. "I (Vang Chou) flew closer to see at least three 50-caliber machine guns. I radioed again to Ly Lue (another Hmong pilot) to tell him I had more than trucks; I had an NVA gun position … ."

I flew low over the NVA gun positions one more time. Midway in my second pass, machine gun fire burst through the plane, up through my body, through my right arm, through my chest, through the windshield. Blood and flesh spattered Sam and the cockpit control panel. Stunned but conscious, I realized I was critically wounded. I was bleeding heavily from my mouth.

With the wind howling through the ragged hole in the windshield, not knowing the extent of the plane's damage, I told Sam to shoot all the smoke rockets. After he fired the rockets, Sam managed to find two morphine tablets for me.

Sam was scared. We were both covered with blood. Sam took over the controls and radioed Cricket. "We've been hit! My man General Direction is critical!" Cricket responded, "Can you make it to Korat? There's a hospital there." I knew Korat was more than two hours from our position. I shouted to Sam over the noise of the wind. "No! Not Korat! No gas! Too far! I can't make it to Korat! Take me to Sam Thong." The American voice from Cricket said, "OK, do as he wants." With the cover of two Skyraiders, Sam flew Vang Chou and the damaged aircraft to Sam Thong, where massive blood transfusions and surgery kept him alive.

Events like this were common during the civil war in Laos. The spotter pilots knew there was a competent and caring American physician at Sam Thong who would take good care of them. Wounded pilots were brought into Sam Thong on a regular basis. In fact, Robert records a spotter pilot story in his letters:

9/14/66 — About 12:30 p.m., Charlie Jones, Captain John Lee (recently arrived from England), and Al Schwartz, a Porter pilot, were spotting targets for the T-28 jets only about five miles from here when ground fire hit their plane. One bullet passed through Schwartz's right foot and grazed Charlie's wrist. The pilot was able to bring the plane in and land it here. His injury was a rather deep laceration of his right instep area. It was no real problem to repair. He should do OK. Before he left the hospital, his friends from Site 10-A sent over a sealed envelope. Inside was a big, cardboard Purple Heart. He really appreciated their gesture. The same pilot had three planes shot down in Korea. He told me that he knew I was here and would take real good care of him. I really appreciated his confidence. This type of incident really brings the war close to home, especially when someone you know really well gets hurt. (By way of explanation — the protocol set by General Vang Pao and Air America called for an Air America pilot and a Hmong spotter to fly in a slow fixed-wing plane over enemy territory to spot their locations. Then Hmong pilots who had been trained by the US Air Force would arrive in T-28 jets to bomb the enemy locations. The Hmong pilots proved to be courageous and relentless in protecting their homeland.)

Then in another incident, Captain Jackson flew out to the scene of an air crash to care for one of Pop Buell's main men. His willingness to not only provide excellent emergency care but also fly with the patient to an advanced care hospital further cemented his reputation as a doctor who cared deeply and would "go the extra mile":

9/15/66 — I am writing this letter from Udorn. There was a Helio crash early this morning near our hospital. I was flown out to the crash scene and found the pilot with second- and third-degree burns of his face, neck, arms, and hands. A native was riding in the right front seat and had third degree burns over 50 percent of his body. They were brought back here, cleaned up, and dressed. I did a tracheotomy on the Laotian co-pilot. He is one of Pop's head men, so it was decided to air-evacuate him to Korat Army Hospital. I flew with him to Udorn in a Helio, then transferred to a twin-engine Beechcraft to fly him to Korat. The patient made the trip OK.

With incidences like the above, Robert's status as a "celebrity" at Sam Thong began. Pilots and ground troops began to hear of the excellent care by the American doctor. He also encountered multiple colorful and influential personalities in Laos, including Pop Buell.

A retired farmer from Steuben County, Indiana, Edgar "Pop" Buell joined International Voluntary Services, the precursor to the Peace Corps, after his wife's death in 1958 at the age of forty-seven. (For those interested, you may watch an archived documentary on Pop Buell by Walter Cronkite listed in Resources). Hoping to improve quality of life, IVS volunteers served in third-world countries with a focus on Vietnam and Laos from 1963-1972. Before the Vietnam War heightened, Pop Buell earned the confidence and trust of the Hmong people as he carried out his primary responsibility of agricultural advisor, and as he lived among them "in a hut without plumbing or electricity." This reminded him of "growing up on the farm in Indiana." Eventually, he worked for USAID in Sam Thong, where he organized relief aid to the Hmong refugees and highlanders fleeing the Communist Pathet Lao and assisted CIA efforts to support the Hmong. While the "United States sent more than 500,000 soldiers to Vietnam, only a few Americans — both civilian and military — worked in Laos." In a *Newsday* article in 1967, author John Steinbeck remarked during a visit to Laos: "I think Pop is an example of how the ancient gods were born ... Whether you believe it or not, there are still giants in the earth." An indication of Pop Buell's valuable work on behalf of the CIA, the Hmong, and the refugees: The Communists put him on a "hit list," resulting in his urgent departure from Laos in 1974 prior to the fall of Saigon in 1975.

Two months after Robert arrived at Sam Thong, Pop Buell walked up to him one late afternoon after Robert had completed a grueling day of surgery. "Captain, I have a proposition for you." With obvious excitement in his voice, Pop announced, "You and I are just alike. We both grew up on a farm. We are both accustomed to the privations of this place. I can tell that you have a genuine love for these mountain people — same as I do. It springs from our common Christian upbringing. I serve these people with a missionary zeal. Doc, it's the same spiritual motivation that I perceive to be in your heart." He paused, gathered his breath, looked straight into Robert's eyes and spoke earnestly, "You and I work well together. We are two peas in a pod. More than that, the people here appreciate and respect both of us. I want to ask you to come back here when your military obligation is over. This place is perfect for you. Not many stateside physicians would survive here, but you actually thrive here. Would you just pray about it?"

Robert was taken aback. As much as he loved the medical work, he had never considered staying longer than his tour or even coming back. He stared intently at Pop through his bushy eyebrows, then breaking into a wide smile, he responded, "Pop, you have been here too long. You're daffy if you think I'm going to stay away from Abbot and my kids one day longer than I have to." With that he turned and walked quickly away, high-stepping through the red mud.

Pop just stared after him, obviously disappointed.

Pop repeated the invitation two and half weeks later, per Robert's letter to Abbot on September 25, 1966:

Pop again asked me tonight if I had arranged for you and the children to come over here. He said he would start my house right away, a two-story one. He gets really peeved when I just tell him he must be crazy. It would be a nice experience, but the hardship and potential hazard would be too much for you. Also, no white married woman has ever been allowed to stay up here with her family.

It didn't take long for Robert's strong work ethic, medical competence, and genuine compassion to impress other influential players in Laos, including the commanding officers who began to notice his accomplishments. He received multiple commendations for his medical service in Laos. His letter records on July 27, 1966:

Colonel Brannon, the 7th Air Force Command surgeon from Saigon, and Colonel Pettigrew, the Air Attaché here in Laos, visited today. I took Colonel Brannon (he is an orthopedist) on rounds, as most of our cases are orthopedic. He was generally well-pleased with the type of care given, and he commended me on my work. I was afraid he would say something about my beard, but he did not.

Then on August 3, 1966:

Another big wheel was here today. Dr. Tirsh (Colonel), the commander of the 17th Army Field Hospital, came to Sam Thong hospital today. He, too, was real impressed with the hospital set-up and the work being done.

Later on August 24, 1966:

I just flew back to Site 20 from the nearby city where I attended a party for Major Keeler at Colonel Pettigrew's. I met several of my old buddies from Udorn who were recently sent up here to work. I was overwhelmed by the light in which the people here (Air Force people, especially Colonel Pettigrew) hold me because of my work at the hospital. To hear them talk, I'm the best doctor in the country. I just try to do a good job, and evidently word has trickled down to them about the work we do up here.

Robert was not only noticed by the American military personnel and Pop Buell with USAID but also by the Laotian military. At one time, General Ma, the head of the Laotian Air Force, became quite ill. There were many options for medical doctors in Laos that he could have called upon, both Laotian and American military, but he sent for Captain Jackson at Sam Thong, whose reputation for diagnosing and treating malaria properly had spread throughout the small country. Robert wrote regarding the incident on September 22, 1966:

> I was called to Udorn today to see General Ma, the head of the Laotian Air Force. He had been sick for a week with chills, fever, and today had a blackout spell. Udorn is the provincial capital city of Laos and is where the king lives. It is located up North on the Mekong River. It is sixty air miles north of here.

There is no mention of General Ma's diagnosis or treatment plan, but he survived to command the Laotian Air Force for many more years.

Robert continued to be surprised by the high-level people who took notice of his work in Sam Thong. His diary on October 2, 1966, says:

> I met the ambassador to Laos, Mr. Sullivan, while in Vientiane this weekend. He was very nice and immediately commented on the report I wrote about the hospital in August. I was surprised he had gotten a copy or even remembered it.

The quality and importance of the work in Sam Thong was noticed by this American ambassador to Southeast Asia. However, it really is no surprise that Mr. Sullivan remembered Captain Jackson's report about Sam Thong, because, as time has passed, it became apparent that others called the secret war in Laos "William Sullivan's war." "There wasn't a bag of rice dropped in Laos that [Sullivan] didn't know about," observed Assistant Secretary of State William Bundy. According to author William Leary, "The CIA was largely responsible for conducting military operations in Laos, but the US Ambassador was the man in charge." Nevertheless, it amazed the captain that of all the reports that crossed Sullivan's desk regarding a war-torn part of the world, he would recall Robert's report about the work at his little hospital in the remote mountains of Laos.

Captain Jackson also interfaced with the charismatic Laotian, General Vang Pao, whose role in Laos is summarized in the follow excerpt:

> Vang Pao commanded a secret army of his mountain people in a long, losing campaign against Communist insurgents. Large portions of the Ho Chi Minh trail, the serpentine route used by North Vietnam to funnel supplies southward, ran through Laotian territory. The United States wanted to interdict the supply route, rescue American pilots shot down over Laos, and aid anti-Communist forces in the continuing civil war. The CIA recruited General Vang Pao for the job and supported his Hmong army for more than ten years. General Vang Pao organized 7,000 guerrillas initially, then steadily increased the force to 39,000, leading them in many successful battles, often against daunting odds. William Colby, CIA director in the mid 1970s, called him the "biggest hero of the Vietnam War." When the CIA approached General Pao in 1960, he was already fighting Laotian Communists. The next year, he also fought Communists from Vietnam after they crossed the Laotian border. The CIA did not command the general's army at any level because his pride and temper never permitted it.

Robert was often invited with other officers to attend the celebrations at General Pao's headquarters across the valley from Sam Thong at Site 90. One such event was described in his letter dated July 30, 1966, in the previous chapter when he attended a *basi* at General Vang Pao's headquarters.

General Vang Pao led troops into combat personally and was known to declare, "If we die, we die together. Nobody will be left behind." As an active participant against Communist insurgency, General Pao incurred wounds multiple times as he led his Hmong warriors into battle. In late September 1966, he was wounded yet again and required surgery in Hawaii on his arm. He returned to Laos with a physical therapist named Skip Dayton, whom Robert hoped to utilize for therapy with his own patients in Sam Thong.

In late October 1966, a chopper landed on the dirt airstrip close to the San Sook Hospital at Sam Thong. As usual, when he was not in surgery, Robert ran out to the chopper to help offload and triage the wounded. To his astonishment, the first one off the chopper was none other than General Vang Pao himself, who immediately came to attention. Robert stopped in his tracks, came to attention himself, and gave the general a smart salute. Returning his salute, the general pointed into the chopper and spoke in heavily accented English, "Doctor, please, my colonel. He have serious head wound." The distress on his face was plainly evident. Looking into the interior of the helicopter, Robert saw a wounded man bearing a colonel's insignia lying on a stretcher with a profusely bleeding scalp wound. He had been accidentally shot in the head by a signal flare, badly lacerating his scalp and rendering him unconscious. He was just beginning to slowly regain his senses while blood continued to flow from the open wound.

Taking charge immediately, Robert commanded, "Quickly. Help me take him to the OR." The general stood aside as his soldiers carried the wounded colonel into the operating room. The colonel's head was shaved, prepped, and an extensive laceration repaired in short order. Robert looked up once to behold the general, multiple of his staff members, and four bodyguards with submachine guns observing his surgical technique. When Robert finished, the patient sat on the side of the bed, groggy, but all patched up. General Vang Pao and his staff were all smiles. Captain Jackson's celebrity status continued to escalate!

Long before the French or American military arrived in Southeast Asia and long after they left, missionaries made their way to Indochina, as that part of the world was previously designated. Called by God, this army of men and women served the people by providing medical care, education, and instruction in agriculture techniques. More than anything, they were called to preach the Good News of Jesus Christ to people groups that were Buddhists, animists, or ancestor worshipers. One such individual was Don Scott, whom Robert wrote about on August 1, 1966:

I had a nice visit with Don Scott, a Christian church missionary, who works this area. His family lives in Vientiane. His members here just completed a church. The roof is of tin and the walls are made of used gasoline drums that have been split in half and flattened out. He walked five hours to get a helicopter to come and pick up a sick child and bring him to the hospital.

And again on August 8, 1966:

The head nurse [at Sam Thong hospital], Miss Cheri, is a Christian and attends the little Christian church run by Don Scott, the Canadian missionary. I am going to get a hymnal from Udorn and together we will try to teach some hymns to the other nurses, and maybe eventually start a little service each Sunday morning.

When I spoke with Don Scott, he was living in retirement in Canada. He said to me, "One of the things I recall most vividly was the interest of the military doctors in the primary health needs of the village people. They were more than willing to show me how to give injections when necessary. The most common illnesses were malaria, hepatitis, stomach parasites, and skin rashes. I remember the military doctors making up a medical kit for me that I could carry as I walked to the various villages. Inevitably, when I would arrive, people would come to me for help with their ailments. Most of the time, I would dispense oral medicines for malaria and parasites. However, the most common request was for the kind of medicine that had to be injected! People often wanted Vitamin B by injection. They insisted that nothing was as good as getting a shot! They often complained they didn't have strength if they didn't get a shot.

"It was quite an experience tramping the trails in northern Laos during those years of the Vietnam War. We faced constant attacks from the Pathet Lao army (the Communist faction of the tripartite government of Laos). The doctors at Sam Thong were desperately needed to help the Hmong army, who, under the leadership of General Vang Pao, were holding back the Communist forces trying to control northern Laos. I often required his permission to walk into various areas where a number of Christian villages were isolated from the Christian community in the countryside. There had been a spiritual awakening in the midst of the Hmong in the mid-1950s to the early 1960s. Tens of thousands of Hmong had come to faith in Jesus Christ during that time. Entire villages had converted to Christianity. On occasion, I had the privilege to preach God's Word to as many as 1,500 Hmong believers at one time. It was an amazing time!

"Once, I walked into the town of Long Tiene and was immediately confronted by a group of US military advisors who demanded to know what this six-foot-three-inch tall, blond-haired Canadian was doing walking around alone in a war zone! When I informed them who I was and what I was about, we became fast friends. They made me their honorary chaplain and invited me to pray over their missions, which often involved great risk. I worked as a missionary with the Christian and Missionary Alliance in Laos from 1964-1969. I was evacuated from Saigon at the end of

April 1975 on a Canadian Air Force plane that came to Saigon to evacuate the Canadian Embassy staff at the closing of the embassy."

Having grown up in a Southern Baptist church, Robert had been imbued with an interest in foreign missions. No doubt he had heard many stories of Baptist missionaries in far-flung parts of the world like Lottie Moon, a Baptist missionary in China for over forty years. The annual Southern Baptist mission offering collected every year at Christmas is named after Lottie Moon. I have no doubt that Robert had a sincere interest in cooperating with these missionaries in sharing the gospel with the Laotian people. Lottie Moon would have been proud!

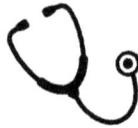

17

NUMBER ONE HAS LEFT THE AREA

After five months in the north country, Robert was three weeks away from his scheduled departure for his home in the United States. He had participated in four-to-five major surgeries per day, flown in more than ninety combat missions in enemy territory, visited dozens of remote villages on humanitarian medical missions, participated in search-and-rescue missions for downed American pilots, established a much-needed blood donor program for the San Sook Hospital, and immensely improved relations with the indigenous Laotian people. He thoroughly enjoyed gaining the surgical experiences and making the acquaintances of Pop Buell, General Vang Pao, and all of his military compatriots like Bob Kosha, John Reid, and Colonel Charles Ramsey.

Constant danger existed from enemy attack, from being hit by ground fire while flying combat missions or actually being shot down. In fact, the Viet Cong overran the Sam Thong hospital and airstrip in 1970 — four years after Robert left — leaving behind satchel charges to ultimately explode, and causing the hospital to burst into flames, destroying it completely. All of the hospital personnel, USAID personnel and schoolteachers fled into the surrounding hillside.

Nevertheless, a greater danger lurked in the Southeast Asian jungle — a danger greater than bullets, bombs or booby traps. The most dangerous animal in the world roamed quite freely in Laos, as indeed it did in all of Southeast Asia and many other countries — the mosquito. Why was it so dangerous? "The female Anopheles mosquito can carry malaria, an infectious disease caused by five plasmodium parasites. Among these, the *P. falciparum* and *p. vivax* parasites pose the greatest threat to humans when bitten and transmitted by an infected mosquito. Malaria is an acute febrile illness occurring ten-fifteen days after the bite. The first symptoms — fever, headache, and chills — may be mild and difficult to recognize as malaria, but if not treated within twenty-four hours, the *p. falciparum* malaria can progress to severe illness, multiple organ failure, and even death. Children under five years of age are the most vulnerable group affected by the disease; in 2019, children accounted for 67 percent (274,000 of the 409,000 malarial deaths worldwide)." In the 1960s-1970s during the Vietnam War, approximately 500,000 people died annually worldwide from malaria. Dad's diary substantiated the prevalence of malaria among children in Laos, since many of his patients with malaria were infants and children.

Robert and his military friends slept under mosquito nets every night, but that didn't protect him on the rural visits to care for the mountain people. One week after one such visit, his situation changed dramatically on November 23, 1966, when he contracted cerebral *(falciparum)* malaria, the very condition that he and Dr. K. treated every day in their medical clinic. His diary entry for November 23 reads, "Too sick to write tonight. Had high fever and chills. Possible malaria or jungle fever. Unless you hear something different, I should be OK in a day or so."

That was optimistic thinking, because the next seven days were definitely touch and go for the good doctor, as he suffered with a high fever, dehydration, delirium, hallucinations and — incredibly — a loss of forty pounds in those seven days. The military doctors feared the worst — that he would not survive.

On Thanksgiving Day, November 24, all of Sam Thong gathered on the clay runway to watch as their beloved American doctor was carried by stretcher to a Porter to be flown to Udorn Air Force Base. There were grave expressions on the faces of the medical personnel. The Laotian nurses whom he had helped to train wept silently. Everyone understood that when American personnel contracted *falciparum* malaria, they were shipped out — never to return. They often did not survive.

The Porter lifted off with their favorite American doctor inside, flew in long slow circles until it reached 9,000 feet, enough to clear the surrounding mountaintops, and then disappeared toward the south. Number One had left the area for the last time.

The following are other diary entries for the week:

November 22, 1966 — Overall aching, muscle pain, chills all night. Started on Aralen (chloroquine — malaria treatment drug) and aspirin.

November 23, 1966 — Bed all day. No appetite. Chills and fever. Felt very bad. No sleep Wednesday night.

November 24, 1966 — Thanksgiving. Feel like dying. Fainted on getting up. 2:00 p.m. Decide to fly to Udorn. Unable to eat, dyspnea. Flown to Udorn in Porter. Carried to plane on stretcher. All of Sam Thong witnesses my departure. Bad feeling I will not be back. Gave instructions to Bob (Kosha) regarding my goods. Arrived Udorn at 4:30 p.m. Taken by ambulance to dispensary. Felt like hell. Two or three doctors check me — malaria smear positive for *falciparum*. I have really had a setback emotionally. Had hoped for dengue. Now know I must leave Thailand for treatment at Clark. Spent Thursday night at Udorn dispensary — very uncomfortable.

November 25, 1966 — Awake early. Small breakfast. Feel some better. Colonel Ramsey came by — he will ship my goods home to States. In afternoon, began to have chills. Feel worse than ever. Delirious. Feel like dying for sure — doctors concerned. I thrash about the bed — have periods of stupor. IV (with quinine added) started. Plan for air evacuation for Clark made. Will leave around

6:30. Colonel Ramsey back to see me. I became upset and want to cry. I felt so very bad, really thought this was my last day on earth. Had seen too much malaria.

Colonel Ramsey received a call at his Udorn headquarters that Robert would soon leave for Clark airbase in the Philippines and had an urgent need to see him. When Ramsey arrived, Robert was highly upset, believing he was just a few hours from death. Ramsey recalled:

> He was sick, and it scared the hell out of me. He was as sick as anyone I had ever seen that wasn't shot to pieces or burned to a crisp, and Bob [Robert] knew it. It was quite a few hours before the aircraft was leaving, so I stayed with him the whole time he was there. He was like one of my kids then, and I sat and held his hand. We talked when he felt like it, but he never let go of my hand for hours. He kept saying, "Colonel, I'm not going to make it. They still need me. What are Abbot and the kids going to do? I should have stayed home. Will you see that they are all right? Please go and talk to them for me and tell them I am sorry. I should have stayed at home."
>
> I sat there almost all of the night and held Bob's [Robert's] hand and talked to him, but mostly listened and prayed a little, successfully I guess, because God doesn't always let the good die young, at least not too young.

After Ramsey left, Robert was placed on a stretcher to board the flight to Clark. He was "doped up with 100 mg of Demerol."

November 25, 1966 journal entry continued — Put in plane — only stretcher case was me. Hundred milligrams of Demerol had me doped. Trip real sketchy. Mouth dry from panting breath.

Feels raw. Terrible headache. Cannot sleep. Everyone on plane keeps looking suspiciously at me. Do not remember landing at Clark but remember being carried into a long ward filled with beds. No patients there but me. IV still going. Asked for aspirin for headache. Dr. Montgomery checks me around 11:00 p.m. Very fitful night. Headache, chills, fever, very little sleep. IV beginning to hurt. Had to be changed.

November 26, 1966 — Still delirious. No appetite, not even for drinking. Visited by Dr. George Grinnan, Gunter (AFB) classmate. Very happy to see him. Too weak to talk to him. Drifting into stuporous state. Aching headache all day. Slight improvement Saturday night. Got in wheelchair for trip to telephone. Called Abbot. So nice to hear her voice and reassure her with tongue in cheek. Fall back to bed — no strength. If ever I needed you, it is now. Please pray for me.

November 27, 1966 — IV stopped. Thank goodness — still unable to eat. Beginning to have hallucinations — especially when eyes are closed. See many varied sights, all in color, duck under pillow to get away from wild bulls. Tried to stay awake and ward off hallucinations. Three ugly wash women beat me with mops. I am scared to shut my eyes. Dr. Grinnan back by — he later told me he thought I was going crazy. I was worried, too. Fever began to go down Sunday night. George Grinnan takes over case Sunday. Decides not to fly me to Japan. Call Abbot Sunday night — a little better — maybe.

November 28, 1966 — Moved to ward 12. Very weak — little fever, no appetite. Sleep most all day.

November 29, 1966 — Took first shower. Feel better. Appetite coming around. Spleen still palpable. Started on Dapsone for three days, along with quinine po (by mouth).

November 30, 1966 — Continue to improve. Out to supper

with Dr. Grinnan and wife Maryanne. Very nice. Real good people.

December 1, 1966 — Improving. Still big spleen. Sleep most of day. Movie on ward that night.

December 2, 1966 — Started to read today. Stopped at 6:30. No fever. Feel good. Out to supper with George and Maryanne. In at 10:00 p.m.

December 3, 1966 — Up early. Good breakfast. To BX (Base Exchange) and shop for one hour. Back to reading, finished two more books. Plan to leave Monday for States.

As he had promised Abbot, he was able to make it home for Christmas, but there was no opportunity for a *basi* for Number One before he left Sam Thong! Nevertheless, a huge celebration occurred in the Jackson household because our Number One Dad had arrived home safely! When he entered our home, he bowed at the waist, folded his hands in front of his face and said, *"Sah bah dee"* — the typical Laotian greeting, and a habit that he maintained for years after returning home.

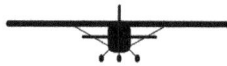

18

AIR FORCE LIFE AFTER LAOS

"Is there a doctor in the arena?" The urgent query sounded again over the PA system: "Is there a doctor in the arena?" We heard this message at a rodeo near our home in Alexandria, Louisiana. The arena was just two streets over from where we lived on Hall Street. I hung out at the arena as an eleven-year-old boy fascinated by the bucking horses and Brahma bulls. They even had sheep, which I had never seen in real life back in South Carolina.

Our family was present at a rodeo when the announcement blared over the loudspeaker. To the dismay of the crowd, a bull rider had just been thrown and then gored severely. The entire audience gasped in concert as the bull hoisted him off the ground and suspended him briefly in the air on his horns. With his massive head, he threw the wounded and bleeding rider to the ground. In an instant, Dad jumped up and rushed down the steps. He vaulted the railing, landed on the arena floor, and in ten steps arrived alongside the injured bull rider. That's when the PA system crackled with a request for a physician. The doctor in the house was already at the side of the injured rider before the announcement could even be made. Quickly, Dad assessed the rider's injuries, and someone called an ambulance. Before long, it arrived — and off they went to the hospital, with Dad unsurprisingly in the rear of the ambulance. The rodeo continued as usual and we departed for home without our doctor dad. He eventually caught a ride back from the hospital in another ambulance with yet another story to tell.

Due to the potentially grave consequences if he should contract malaria a second time, military doctors denied Dad's request to return to his post at Sam Thong. Therefore, he completed his remaining one-year obligation to the Air Force at England Air Force Base in Alexandria, where he became the chief medical officer at the base infirmary. The entire family had moved with him this time and lived off base temporarily near the arena until on-base housing was available. All of the children enrolled in school, and our family joined Parkview Baptist Church — a delightful Christian home for us, as the congregation embraced our family and loved us well. During our short time at Parkview, Dad immediately became a leader — heading up a building fund effort. I remember being a part of their RAs (Royal Ambassadors) group, which traveled to Oklahoma City one summer for the annual RA congress, where I studied world missions with thousands of other Baptist youth from all over the US. We camped out beside a river at night and listened to missionaries describe their exploits during the daytime conferences.

The celebrity status he attained in Laos continued, partly because of his oratorical skill in describing his experiences in Southeast Asia and partly because of his exceptional accomplishments in SEA — for which he was voted Flight Surgeon of the Year for the Tactical Air Command in 1966. Having taken note of his stellar accomplishments in SEA, the Air Force awarded him multiple, significant commendations in rapid succession — including the Joint Service Commendation Medal for his "meritorious service with the Joint United States Military Advisory Group in Thailand," the Airman's Medal for "heroism involving voluntary risk of life at a forward operating strip within Southeast Asia," the Air Medal for "meritorious achievement for participating in sustained aerial flight as a combat crew member," and the Legion of Merit for "exceptional merito-rious conduct in performance of outstanding service to the United States as physician and surgeon to friendly indigenous forces in a highly critical area of Southeast Asia." The explanation of this last award said: "Captain

Jackson's professional competence, astute leadership, and exemplary initiative contributed greatly to the encouragement of the native peoples' resistance to aggression, as well as to the morale of the indigenous troops. The superior initiative, outstanding professionalism, and personal endeavor displayed by Captain Jackson reflect great credit upon himself and the United States Air Force." Not to be forgotten, the Bronze Star Medal was mentioned previously. As you can tell, each of these commendations references Southeast Asia, but not Laos, since his involvement there was top secret for many years.

After his return from Southeast Asia, Robert became a popular speaker for the Tactical Air Command and the Air Commandos, promoting the war effort and recruiting other MDs to volunteer for duty in Sam Thong rather than merely accepting cushy assignments behind the lines. Asked to speak often and motivated by his patriotic fervor, he took every opportunity to educate as many as would listen by sharing his slides about his six-month tour in Laos — although he could only describe his location as a jungle hospital in Southeast Asia, since his involvement there was considered top secret for years afterwards.

In his practice prior to military service, Dad rarely had more than a day or two off at a time due to the demands of his busy private medical practice — late hours, frequent ER duty, and the ever-present responsibility of delivering babies. In contrast, Air Force life (post-Southeast Asia) afforded him more time off to spend with his family than he had ever enjoyed before, with eight-to-five office hours and only occasional weekend duties. We bowled as a family. He and Mom played golf. Having already obtained his pilot's license, Dad perfected his flying skills in the afternoons, while Mom took a few more flying lessons (after her initial lessons in Sumter, South Carolina, while Dad was in Southeast Asia). She came close to flying solo for her license but never followed through. She didn't want to compete with the jets at England AFB, but Mom recalls one flying lesson there. Using her South Carolina, Lowcountry southern drawl, she spoke into her mic to the air traffic controller, "This is Novemba-Ninah, Ninah, Fowah, Fowah, Seven requestin' permission to take awf on runway three-fowah."

The ATC immediately responded in a fake drawl, "Can you pu-leease say that agayun?" She heard peals of laughter on the other end. Fear of the jets, and a little bit of embarrassment, effectively ended her flying lessons.

Our family participated in the many activities scheduled by the Officer's Club, including a gala where Mom pantomimed "Annie Get Your Gun," wearing my sister Anne's western outfit. We traveled to New Orleans on at least one occasion and took an extended two-week vacation — our first and only two-week vacation — in the southwestern United States. We visited the ruins of the Pueblo Indians, Carlsbad Caverns, the Grand Tetons, the Old Faithful Geyser, and Jackson Hole, Wyoming, with four kids and a beagle in the back of a station wagon pulling a pop-up camper.

Robert was quite tempted to stay in the Air Force and take one of several choice assignments offered to him. However, the call of home, his patients, and his extended family appealed to his sense of family and responsibility. We left for our home in Manning in February 1968, but prior to our departure, we attended Parkview Baptist one final time. I remember vividly that last Sunday at the church. Someone asked my dad to pray during the service; in the middle of his prayer, he became emotional and wept aloud as he thanked God for the people in that church who had ministered to our family. I am sure he was full of conflicting emotions in his heart as he contemplated leaving a loving church family, the ease of stateside Air Force life, and the many good friends he had made at the church as well as at the base.

During the trip home to South Carolina, we encountered an unusual winter storm in Mississippi. A moving company had loaded our large household goods in its truck while we stuffed our personal belongings into a canvas cartop carrier, and the whole "kit and caboodle" was ready to go. Each of us left Louisiana with mixed emotions; nevertheless, we headed home with eager anticipation. After traveling for a while, that eagerness turned to anxiety, as all of us noticed the heavy sleet beginning to fall, along with the temperatures. Nightfall arrived, enveloping the interstate in a deep darkness — although the white blanket of snow on the surrounding countryside reflected the headlights of passing cars. The roads grew more treacherous. Dad slowly and carefully navigated the ice-covered roadway, but no one thought about our personal belongings in the luggage ensconced safely — or so we thought — in the cartop carrier.

Suddenly, we heard and felt the sleet-covered luggage carrier lift off the roof of our station wagon. Horrified, we looked behind us, only to see it struck immediately by a following vehicle. Suitcases exploded, releasing our clothing, personal items, and important documents. The sleet-laden wind and passing vehicles blew our belongings haphazardly all over the interstate. While Mom stayed in the car with the younger children, Dad and I scampered around for thirty minutes in the freezing sleet, collecting the suitcases and clothes, and chasing windblown papers. A couple of cars stopped, and the drivers got out to help. One deceitful helper purloined a small blue suitcase carrying Mom's jewelry and gifts from Thailand — much to her chagrin and never-ending regret. What a sad conclusion to a joyful and meaningful last year in the Air Force!

Although our trip home ended on a note of frustration and sadness, my dad's two-year stint in the Air Force was filled with adventure, new friends, and a delightful family experience. Now it was time to turn his heart toward home — back to the extended family that he dearly loved, back to his patients who desperately missed him, and back to the sandy soil of Clarendon County where his bare feet once ran carefree.

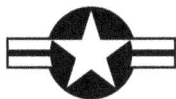

19

THE PATRIOT

Even in high school, Robert Jackson exhibited a patriotic zeal, delivering a speech as president of the student body entitled "Peace with Freedom." Perhaps this was inspired by the exemplary military service of his older brother Jimmy, a decorated Army veteran of World War II, and his brother Ralph who served in the Korean Conflict. Ralph graduated from Clemson College in 1950 as a first lieutenant. One year later, he was a company commander in Korea, where he served for two years, mostly on the front lines. An expert rifleman and instructor in 30-caliber and 50-caliber machine guns, he received two Bronze Stars for bravery in combat, but his family states he shared few details of his exploits while in Korea. Obviously, Robert had much to live up to and much to fuel the flames of his patriotic fervor.

Robert attended Clemson College during the year Clemson transitioned from a military school to a civilian school (1955). The Cadet Corps no longer existed; nevertheless, every male student was still required to participate in ROTC during their first two years of school. Wearing an ROTC uniform, Robert marched in formation with all the other male students on Bowman Field in front of Tillman Hall.

Robert's patriotic fervor removed any reluctance about his personal involvement in the military — and, ultimately, his assignment in Southeast Asia. Once inducted, Robert loved all things military. He embraced the order and structure of the US Air Force, which suited his personality perfectly. Robert always strived for excellence in everything in which he was involved, explaining why he quickly rose to the top even in the military — as evidenced by his numerous citations and awards. His enthusiasm, friendliness and leadership skills caused him to be a leader among men. This was true of him in his civilian, medical and military life.

An insight into Robert's strong, patriotic beliefs is found in a diary entry from Southeast Asia, sandwiched between a description of the daily surgeries and his bi-weekly flights to Udorn to pick up donated blood.

> Diary entry 10/6/66 —
>
> No surgery today, other than inserting a chest tube to drain an empyema of the right pleural cavity. A few minor wounded came in, but nothing serious. I do not mind the service, except for the separation from you and the children. *I feel that each healthy American male should serve his country in the armed forces for a two-year period. Some, of necessity, must sacrifice more than others in separation from their loved ones, enduring hardships and even suffering physical hurt, but this is the price of liberty as we know it in the US, and I am proud to be able to contribute a part to preserving the heritage and freedom enjoyed by all Americans. I am proud to be an American over here. My every thought and action is done so as to reflect our good will and reinforce the principles of freedom as we know them. Those back in the States who would defame our flag, criticize our nation's policies, rebuke the draft, disobey the law, disrupt peaceful neighborhoods, violently attack our Constitution, and forget individual rights and prerogatives have certainly forgotten their heritage, or perhaps they have never realized the impor-tance of national solidarity. I wish there was some way to impress the youth of America the importance of freedom, liberty, and a true pursuit of happiness — happiness which is only possible*

through a strong, armed force to preserve the peace and protect the homeland. Maybe in time the Beatnik [a term associated with non-conformism and drug use] *population, rebellious young people, and critics of our foreign policy will realize that a strong United States is necessary to preserve our priceless freedom. When this realization occurs, then certainly our national effort will be greatly enhanced.* [The italics and bold type are preserved from his original letter.] I go to Udorn in the morning to pick up the bi-weekly blood donated for use here at the hospital.

Growing up, I often observed my father standing at attention with eyes focused on the flag during the Pledge of Allegiance and the singing of "The Star-Spangled Banner" at civic and athletic events. Others in the crowd might be talking or moving about, but not my dad. He was intentionally reverential of the flag and that which it represented: liberty, individual rights, and the Constitution — all of which he respected and honored. He also had painful, personal memories of fellow soldiers — both American and Laotian — who gave the last full measure to preserve and protect freedom as evidenced by the following intense monologue I was privileged to hear just prior to a high school football game.

One Friday night when I was in college, I followed my dad to our local high school football game. He was the team physician. After we arrived and walked under the goalposts, "The Star-Spangled Banner" started playing. My dad immediately stood at attention — ramrod straight — with his hand over his heart. Of course, I did the same. I glanced at the stands and noticed people talking and moving about. Dad's eyes were straight ahead and fixed on the flag.

At the conclusion in a moment of candor, he looked at me and said, "Son, that flag represents freedom everywhere in the world." I simply nodded. He continued, "When I was in Southeast Asia, I was often choppered into a remote village on goodwill missions to provide medical care to the Laotian people, who responded with extreme gratefulness. When it was time to leave and my chopper returned to retrieve me, I could see the fear and anxiety in the faces of the people. They never knew if the sound of a chopper represented the North Vietnamese, who killed their old men, kidnapped their young men, and raped their young women — or if it meant the Americans, who brought food, medicine and security. Only when they saw the American flag on the side of the chopper did they relax and smile. Truthfully, I felt the same way. That flag represented freedom."

Then my dad held up his hands in front of him. His lip quivered, but I saw steel in his eyes. "With these hands, I tried to stop the flow of blood of American soldiers — wounded in battle, fighting in a place to which they'd never been and to which they'd never return, for a people they little understood. Nevertheless, they believed in exporting freedom — the same freedom they enjoyed — to other parts of the world. They were willing to bleed and die to liberate oppressed peoples, and they did so proudly under the banner of that flag of freedom. Son, these hands tried to stop the flow of blood of brave, proud American soldiers who called the names of their mothers or their wives before the light went out of their eyes."

He was visibly shaking now as we stood under the goalposts all alone in the glow of the stadium lights. I can see him now, the picture of him in one of his favorite sport coats — yellow in color — seared in my memory. He finished by saying defiantly, "I'll never forget those young soldiers or the oppressed people of Laos. I will always stand tall under that flag. It represents freedom."

About that time, six cheerleaders came running up and stood in a row under the goalposts. We looked up and the home team was on the field, ready to receive the kickoff. I backed up three steps. My dad just grabbed a pompom from one of the cheerleaders and stood there waving a pompom like it was the natural thing to do. Now you know why everybody loved my dad. Now you know why I stand straight at the Pledge of Allegiance and sing loud and proud at the playing of "The Star-Spangled Banner" — the banner that means freedom!

After returning to civilian life, he continued as a sought-after speaker for civic and church groups, describing the war effort and his particular part in that effort. The non-medical part of audiences often had difficulty with his before-and-after medical slides of the wounded soldiers and civilians for whom he and Dr. K. provided such assiduous medical and surgical attention. My cousin Beth reminded me that my father spoke to our Manning High School student body assembly in 1968 — describing his role in Southeast Asia and sharing an edited presentation. I immediately recalled this speech because of the ripples of amazement stirred up among both teachers and students. One of the teachers, May Hinson Jones, was my cousin Beth's aunt on her father's side. Her husband, Bailey Jones, who had become a fast friend of my father's, was on his second tour as a helicopter pilot in Vietnam. He experienced the trauma of his chopper being blown out of the sky and later wrote a book about his Vietnam experience entitled *Year of the Snake: One Helicopter Pilot's Story of a Year in Vietnam's Mekong Delta* (published by Shade Tree Publishers, 1999).

The plight of the American POWs caught the attention of the US public after the hostilities in Southeast Asia ceased — but none more than Dr. Robert Jackson, family doctor in Manning, South Carolina, and former captain in the US Air Force. His heart grieved at the thought of American GIs or pilots being held as political pawns by the North Vietnamese. No doubt they were being treated harshly and deprived of necessary food and medical care. He was filled to the brim with a righteous indignation. Not one to sit idly by, Robert organized events in his hometown to bring attention to the plight of the POWs. He chaired the Week of Concern for POWS and MIAs, and spoke in the schools "where petitions were signed to be delivered to North Vietnamese officials at Paris Peace Talks by Mrs. John C. West, the wife of the governor of South Carolina." I clearly recall being held prisoner with my good friend Larry McCord in an imitation POW camp constructed on the courthouse grounds in downtown Manning and being viewed by hundreds of curious spectators after a parade had processed down Main Street. We all wore POW wristbands with the name of an individual soldier or airman inscribed for whom we all prayed. My dad wrote an endless stream of letters to political personalities, urging them to intervene on behalf of the POWs.

My dad's passionate love for America and her ideals was influenced by his face-to-face encounter with the evils of Communism that not only imprisoned military men, using them as pawns in international negotiations, but also crippled and killed civilians wantonly with bombs, bullets, and land mines in Laos. After the war, the Hmong for whom he cared medically were systematically exterminated by the Communists, using such methods as dropping poisonous chemicals from airplanes on their mountain villages. The love for America and the hatred for Communism burned hot in the heart of this country doctor.

The 1960s and the 1970s were a time of social upheaval in America, with protests against the war, marches on Washington, DC, and burning the flag. Robert had little understanding of draft dodgers and war protesters, and no patience with their perspective. He had seen the evil face of Communism up close and understood clearly that the American way of life was exceptional, unequaled, and superior. For that belief, he made no apology.

Robert's love for the military prompted him to enlist in the Air National Guard in South Carolina, where he was quickly promoted to rank of Major and eventually to Colonel. He continued his designation as Air Surgeon, conducting physicals and health assessments for pilots and all airmen at McEntire Air National Guard Base in Columbia, South Carolina. He flew his own airplane to Columbia once a month (weather permitting) for guard duty, which he thoroughly enjoyed — especially the camaraderie with the pilots and his health clinic medical personnel, many of whom were Vietnam veterans like himself.

He also attended two weeks of training camp each summer. Ron Trotter, a technician in the ANG health clinic, recorded the following incident:

It was a warm, spring day in May 1974, when Dr. Robert Jackson and all of his troops from the 169th TAC clinic reported to the Myrtle Beach AFB Regional Hospital for fifteen days of active duty training. One of the first things we were hit with was that the hospital had scheduled 250 preschool children for physicals over the period of the next three months. "Darling' Doc," as Dr. Jackson was affectionately known by his clinic personnel, thought that this was a gross waste of time and energy. He told the hospital commander that we had come to work and that we would take care of the preschool physicals. The hospital commander agreed with a chuckle and said, "If you think you can, go ahead and do it." Of course, he didn't know about "Darlin' Doc," or the fact that he normally saw sixty-eighty, or more, really sick patients in one day in his medical practice. Two-hundred-fifty preschool physicals in one day? Well, that "twernt nuttin."

Well, he put out the word to the people in scheduling that he wanted all these kids scheduled the following Tuesday at 7:30 a.m. Naturally, they balked but did manage to get them scheduled. On Tuesday morning at 7:30, we were ready — and so were 250 children and their parents all lined up out the hospital door and around the block.

The hospital commander immediately called "Darlin' Doc" in his office and demanded an explanation. "Darlin' Doc" told him in no uncertain terms that we were doing 250 children preschool physicals. The hospital commander said, "There is absolutely no way that you can finish, and if you do you, you will mess up three months of scheduling for the hospital."

"Darlin' Doc" said, "Sorry, but they are already here, and we have already started." At 3:30 that afternoon, the last little one left the hospital with a smile on his face, ready for summer, and for school next fall with his preschool exam behind him and nothing to mess up his summer. "Darlin' Doc" said, "Thanks, folks, for a good job well done. Let's go eat some supper and go to the beach." So ended a day with "Darlin' Doc" and his 169th TAC Clinic.

Why did his medical clinic personnel call him "Darlin' Doc"? In their eyes, their major — their leader — was a man's man. He was hard-driving, aggressive, assertive, and strove for excellence; yet, at the same time, he exhibited kindness, gentleness, and compassion toward his patients. In the male-dominated military world characterized by crudity, cynicism and competition, he was a shining light in the darkness that refused to become like them. He didn't smoke, drink, or curse. He treated others fairly, respectfully, and with kindness. You couldn't rile him or extract from him a critical word. There was no vindictiveness or evidence of a mean streak. Truthfully, Dr. Jackson was a bit of an anomaly, a stark contrast in that jaded, cynical, coarse ex-Vietnam military world. His inner Christian character manifested itself even more brightly in that semidarkness. Out of respect, his medical clinic colleagues referred to him as "Darlin' Doc," a term of affection for the God-fearing, people-loving commanding officer whom they greatly valued.

His responsibility as Air Surgeon in the ANG included flying back seat in the F-102 fighter jets, the jets in service at McEntire in the 1970s. He was required to fly once every ninety days to maintain his status as Air Surgeon. He reveled in that requirement — which he considered more of a thrill and a privilege than a requirement — and flew as often as possible. He often told me that he and his F-102 pilot friends flew to some faraway military base as part of their training requirements, landed, called a cab, and went to eat at a well-known restaurant in town. They then flew back from several states away in forty-five minutes or less in those supersonic jets. Exhilarated by the experience and by the flying time in a jet airplane, this only further fueled his passion for flying, his love for the military, and his love for country — all of which ran hot in his veins. Everyone who knew Robert Jackson can affirm that he was a passionate, patriotic American.

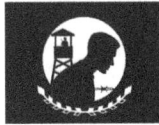

20

THE MAN ON THE VIDEO

"Dr. Jackson, there's an emergency call for you," his nurse reported urgently.

He left an exam room, walked swiftly to his private office, picked up the phone, and answered, "This is Dr. Jackson."

A strained and excited voice came through the line. "Doc, this is J.D. (Daniels). We're at an accident on 95. A tractor-trailer rig rear-ended another large truck and then flipped. We've tried but we can't get the driver out. He's trapped by the collapsed driver's side door. We need your assistance quick-like. The driver's hurt bad."

After obtaining the exact location, Robert was out the back door in a flash. At the time, he drove a baby blue Fairlane 500 Fastback like David Pearson (the NASCAR driver) in which he kept a medical emergency kit at all times. In ten minutes, he arrived at the scene of the accident where he immediately took charge.

Climbing into the cab of the overturned eighteen-wheeler, he assessed the driver's injuries, where he ascertained that the driver was conscious but in significant pain from his trapped left side. Dr. Jackson quickly checked his cervical spine, which was non-tender. His BP was stable and he had no excessive bleeding, so he reassured the driver and began to give instructions for the extrication, which required the assistance of a wrecker driven by Bob Spigner. The wrecker was used to pull the collapsed door away from the driver since no "jaws of life" existed in those days.

189

In another thirty minutes, the driver was freed, placed on a backboard, removed to an ambulance, and taken away to Clarendon Memorial Hospital. The rescue squad members looked around to thank Dr. Jackson, but he was already gone. He had raced back to care for an office full of patients.

After returning from Vietnam, I'm certain Dad missed the challenge of caring for severely injured soldiers and civilians. Well, that didn't last long. We lived on Highway 301 which, until Interstate 95 was constructed, was the major north-south route from New York to Miami, and it ran right through the middle of our rural southern hometown. As you can imagine, many violent vehicular accidents occurred on that road. Our rural hospital was the only medical facility for forty miles in either direction between Florence to the north and Orangeburg to the south. Robert Jackson thrived on being called night or day to attend the scene of a motor vehicle accident anywhere in the county to help extricate the victims and transport them to the hospital, where he would then care for their traumatic injuries. He was a take-charge kind of guy, and he was in his element at the scene of an accident. He was the HMWIC on the scene, which was the military way of saying the "Head Man What's in Charge."

He kept a two-way radio at our home, with an antenna out back that reached halfway to the moon, so he could communicate with any sheriff's deputy anywhere in the county. My sister, Anne, and I became adept at answering that radio, giving his call sign, and taking messages or telling his whereabouts to the ER or sheriff's deputies. My mom used it to tell him to bring home milk or boiled peanuts from Mr. Alsbrooks' grocery store!

My dad was a safety promoter long before the National Transportation Safety Board ever came on the scene. Many years prior to the wearing of seat belts in cars, he promoted them because of all of the vehicular accidents he attended, and because he understood the death and injury that could be prevented. He was such a believer that he had safety belts installed in his automobile long before current laws required them. They stretched across his chest in a big "X" like those used in airplanes. When his brothers saw him in his car with heavy-duty straps crisscrossing his chest, they laughed themselves silly. Not only that, when he went to the scene of an accident, he wore a half helmet like NASCAR drivers wore in those days but with a red cross painted on top. His brothers really howled at that.

For Dad's birthday one year, my uncles gave him a plastic helmet that had a red, rotating light on top as a gag gift. Being the jokester that he was, he loved the gift and kept it in his vehicle. In our small hometown of Manning on the weekends, high schoolers drove from one end of town to the other — from the Bantam Chef restaurant on the south end to Pate's Drive-In Restaurant on the north end. Occasionally on Sunday night after church, Dad loaded all of us kids and Mom in his car. Because he typically replaced his vehicles every two years, he always drove the latest, up-to-date version of some model automobile. It didn't matter. Everyone still recognized Dr. Jackson's car. When there are only 3,000 people in the entire city limits, everyone knows the vehicles of the family doctors in town, even if they changed every two years!

To embarrass my mom and sister, he put that plastic helmet on his head, turned on the rotating light, and "cut" Pate's Drive-In while waving at all the teenagers and adults eating supper after church with his arm hanging out the window. He had to drive slowly through Pate's unpaved parking lot because of deep ruts. We could hear various voices crying out in the darkness, "Hey, Dr. Jackson. Hey, Doc." Mortified, my mom and sister slumped down to the floorboard. My brothers and I just smiled and laughed — enjoying the moment. I think my dad lived for an opportunity to embarrass my mom and sister. Then he made the circuit and repeated this same procedure at the Bantam Chef, while my mother muttered threats from the floorboard. Everybody hollered, "Hey, Dr. Jackson!" They all loved him, and he just smiled and waved at them with that plastic helmet on and the red light rotating. Occasionally, he hit another button and a siren in the helmet sounded off, much to the continued delight of my brothers and me. I always wondered what became of that helmet!

I remember many nights lying in my bed late in the evening — reading (as was my custom) and hearing the two-way radio going off to announce an accident, hearing Dad pound down the hallway and slam the back door, and hearing the roar of his fire-engine-red Pontiac GTO. I then heard the tires squeal as he left our driveway. The big engine emitted a deep throated roar; the tires squealed at each of three turns required to exit our neighborhood. I held my breath until the last tire squeal. Then the silence of our small town returned, and I could hear the crickets outside my open window. I heaved a sigh of relief, smiled, and returned to reading. My doctor dad was going to rescue somebody.

He allowed me to go with him to the scene of an accident once when I was in high school on a black, dark night without any moon or stars. An accident occurred past the turnoff to the Kingstree Highway and halfway to Greeleyville. When we arrived, cars sat on both sides of the road with headlights blinding me, so I couldn't see anything clearly. As we walked quickly to the scene, we found a red Volkswagen perched upside down on the side of the road with a dozen people gathered around. About that time, a grown man let loose a blood-curdling scream, took a breath, and screamed again. I immediately became so nauseated I had to kneel in the tall, wet grass on the side of the road to regain my composure. I was reluctant to go any closer. In fifteen minutes or less, Dad had taken control of the situation, helped extricate the victim, and was back with his assessment: "Broken femur. He'll be fine. We'll meet him at the ER when the rescue squad gets him there. They don't need me here any longer."

Thirty minutes later, we arrived in the ER, where I watched fascinated as he gave the writhing patient morphine, putting him out of his misery. He then drilled a hole in the patient's distal femur, placed a Steinman pin, put him in traction, took an X-ray, and headed home — satisfied that his patient would do well. In today's world, no family doctor would do that — too much liability and no expertise. That patient would have been referred to an orthopedist. Robert Jackson did that every day in Laos. He saw no need in sending the patient to a referral hospital far away from his family. He just handled it. That was a phrase that his employees and the hospital personnel heard him say repeatedly over the years, "We'll just handle it." He did so with confidence and competence.

Before the 1970s, no rescue squad existed in our county. Accident victims arrived at the hospital in private vehicles or hearses owned by funeral homes. Many of them died at the scene or suffered more severe injuries during transport by well-meaning people. In an essay entitled "The Evolution of Rescue Services in Clarendon County" by Carter Jones (at the time of the essay, he was the South Carolina Fire Department historian), he says:

> Hearses served as both funeral coaches as well as ambulances. Beginning around the 1950s, the roofs of hearses could be trans- formed into an emergency vehicle with the quick placement of a Beacon Ray revolving light, which offered minimal visual warning for traffic. Several hearses were installed with small electric sirens that provided some audible signal. None of the hearses carried first-aid equipment, so when a patient was loaded into the back of the ambulance, the patient was on his own until arrival at Clarendon Memorial Hospital. … Rarely any attendants accom- panied the patient.

The volunteer rescue squad eventually purchased a hearse painted orange and white and operated by a few volunteers who often drove it to the scene of an accident. Accident victims, before being loaded into the hearse, looked skeptically at what obviously was a hearse and asked, "Where exactly are we going?" If the victims were not severely injured, they were told tongue-in-cheek, "Depends upon how much money you have." Seeing a need for improvement in this system, Robert Jackson took the initiative to do something. First, he trained a group of volunteers in first aid, CPR, starting IVs, splinting broken bones, applying tourniquets to bleeding extremities, maintaining airways, etc. Then he trained them in the proper techniques for extricating accident victims from vehicles and the use of a backboard to protect the victim's spine. In his essay, Carter Jones reports it like this:

> Around 1965, Dr. Jackson, a local physician and later a Vietnam flight surgeon, approached J.D. Daniels about starting a volunteer rescue squad. Together, these men invited a young attorney, John Land, to meet with them at the Ramada Inn, formerly located at what is now Ram Bay, to discuss the merits of the idea and to proceed with acquiring a state charter ... J.D. Daniels was no stranger to emergency services, because he also served as a volunteer firefighter for the Manning Fire Department for many years and responded to incidents on his own long before rescue became an integral community service.
>
> J.D. and Dr. Jackson held a number of organizational meetings and recruited quite a few local individuals and volunteer firefighters to become charter members of the newly formed Manning rescue squad.
>
> When the rescue squad was initially organized, its mission was primarily focused on rescue and extrication, water search and recovery. A military surplus pickup was equipped with varied rudimentary tools, ropes, jacks, etc. J.D. Daniels owned a large boat that was used in rescue and search operations when drownings occurred, or at times when fishermen were reported missing on the lake.

Dad continued to demonstrate his commitment to training rescue personnel by assisting in instruction for a DHEC-approved EMT training course at Tuomey Hospital in Sumter, South Carolina. Several volunteers from our county, Clarendon, graduated on June 27, 1972. Dad was honored to be the guest speaker and the presenter of their certificates. One of the later volunteers, trained as an EMT and receiving his certification in 1977, was Robert Ridgeway, now a medical doctor himself. He said:

> I worked third shift at Clarendon Memorial Hospital in the beginning. I would be so tired and sleepy in the middle of the night; then, suddenly Dr. Jackson would come bounding through the ER heading to the delivery room. He always walked really fast and always seemed to be wide awake and wide open. He was full of energy and excitement.
>
> Dr. Jackson loved the EMS and on occasion he took the entire group of EMTs to his lake house. He grilled hamburgers for us, then showed us slides of his time in Laos. I was intrigued by the medical slides and his experience. It left a long-lasting impression on me.
>
> Dr. Jackson was always encouraging us to pursue further training and additional education. Because of his encouragement, I went on to paramedic school. My experiences as a paramedic eventually led me to medical school.

Robert Ridgeway graduated from medical school and OB-GYN residency. He served as an OB-GYN in Manning for many years and is now the medical control officer for the Clarendon County Fire Department and EMS.

The rescue squad in Manning still lacked one critical item — a proper rescue vehicle. Dad realized this was an obvious next step, so he once again devised a plan — this time to raise money. Along with a committee of concerned citizens, he organized a community-wide Carolina-Clemson fundraising football game. The idea drew such enthusiasm that all of the local high school and college football talent for a decade clamored to participate. The committee required all of the players to practice and to improve their physical condition for two weeks prior to the game, and, of course, to sign liability waivers in case of injuries.

The game was the talk of the entire county for days, ultimately drawing a huge crowd and raising sufficient funds to purchase the county's first legitimate rescue squad vehicle — including suitable equipment to furnish it. All around, it was a satisfying success — well, except for one part of the story.

As I told you before, Dad always fancied himself to be Terry Bradshaw throwing me the football in the backyard. Since he organized the event, he appointed his brother Scott as coach and arrogated to himself the position of quarterback on the Clemson team. Remember, he was the field general on his high school team. He called the plays, handed off the ball to the running backs, and threw short passes. He performed well until the third quarter when a high school player defensive end clocked him running wide open. He fell to the ground unconscious and didn't wake up for about three minutes. The whole stadium went stone-cold silent. We all thought the new rescue squad vehicle was about to be used for the first time on Dr. Jackson, but he came around and staggered to the sidelines to a big round of applause. My mom gave him the "I told you so" lecture for days afterwards, but we kids were just proud of our dad, even if he did get bulldozed by a high schooler. His brothers never let him live that one down. For years afterwards, whenever the brothers were together, we could hear them say: "Hey, Ralph, you remember the time that high school boy bulldozed Robert at the Carolina-Clemson game?" Then the entire family would rock with laughter — much to Dad's chagrin.

In my interview with Carter Jones, he shared how pleased the rescue squad and later the EMS were with Dad's progressive thinking and willingness to promote new technology:

> We were always thankful for Dr. Jackson's energy, expertise, and vision. He always strived for excellence and progress in medical care in his own medical practice and in our county. While others

were content with things as they were, he was always promoting improvements in patient care and investments in technology. He was selfless with his time, often showing up for search-and-rescue efforts for lost hunters in the woods or lost fishermen on the lake. He was always ready to leave his busy medical practice to help the rescue squad extricate an accident victim from a vehicle on Highway 301 or I-95. I recall multiple incidences where he crawled into a wrecked vehicle to place a cervical collar or correctly position a backboard rather than just giving instructions. I remember seeing him at the scene of an overturned tractor directing the rescue of the unfortunate farmer. I know for a fact that he contributed more than his fair share financially in the early days to secure the survival of our fledgling rescue squad. There was no one quite like Dr. Jackson.

My cousin Beth Hinson phoned me one evening, eager to share yet another emergency situation involving Dad that occurred while she was in high school:

I was sitting at the kitchen table with my uncle Jim and aunt Louise Bennett when we heard a loud automobile crash out on the Jordan Road several hundred yards from their home. I was living with them at the time, caring for my aunt Louise due to her severe rheumatoid arthritis. Both her hands and legs were quite deformed due to the effects of the disease. Uncle Jim and I immediately jumped into his truck and drove out to the Jordan Road where two vehicles, a car and a truck, had collided, with one upside down in the ditch.

There were three high school boys lying in the ditch — two of them moaning and groaning, with one unconscious. Uncle Jim drove back to his house to call the hospital, which then dispatched the county ambulance — a Shelly Brunson Funeral Home hearse. I sat in the ditch, holding the young man who was unconscious and realized that most of the top of his head was missing. The other two continued to complain loudly with their injuries. It became darker and darker as I sat in the ditch with these three seriously injured young men, and I realized there were absolutely no vehicles on the road at that time of night.

I was not aware of it at the time, but Uncle Robert was holding the very first training for the Clarendon County rescue squad that very night. In about thirty minutes, Uncle Robert showed up in his sporty and speedy automobile wearing a white helmet with a red cross on it. He had brought with him all of the trainees from his class. He directed his flashlight at me, surprised to see one of his nieces at the scene of the accident. I immediately said, "Uncle Robert, this one is hurt the worst, and I don't think he's going to make it." He inspected the young man briefly, responding, "Beth, you are right. I don't think he is either." Shortly thereafter, they had loaded all three men into their personal vehicles before the hearse had a chance to arrive and off they went to the hospital. The one young man didn't survive, as we both suspected.

While in my residency program in Spartanburg in 1981, I was in the ER one Saturday night issuing orders to a nurse regarding one of my patients when an EMT stopped and stared at me. Then he smiled and said, "You're the doctor on the videotapes."

I replied, "Excuse me?"

Still smiling, he said, "You're the doctor on the videotapes. You trained me and all of my EMT buddies down in Columbia. Your tapes were excellent training."

I stared at him for a moment; then my little pea-brain clicked, and I responded, "No, sir, that was my father. He trained EMTs by video in the early 1970s. I guess they still use his videos."

He shook my hand and said, "Well, you sure sound like him. I'd recognize that voice anywhere." Then he was gone. I can't tell you how much that warmed my heart to hear that Dr. Robert Jackson's influence still lived on, especially in an area of medicine he dearly loved — emergency medicine.

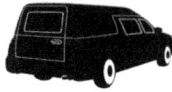

21

MEETING THE NEED

"I'm going to run for sheriff."

Robert's friends looked at him incredulously. "You're going to do what?"

"I'm going to run for sheriff. My older brother Jehu is sheriff in my home county. I have a great deal of respect for him and what he does, so I'm going to run for sheriff."

Robert and his good friend, J.J. Britton, were attending Palmetto Boys' State, a weeklong event designed to introduce the best and brightest high school graduates in South Carolina to the political process. During the week, these young men heard rousing political speeches from various elected officials promoting the civic responsibility of every young American. Mock elections were held during the week between the Red and Blue parties.

J.J. turned and looked at his friends and decided instantly, "Guys, we're going to organize a campaign to promote Robert for sheriff. I am confident he can win."

For several days, they worked vigorously promoting Robert as sheriff of the Red Party. Robert gave a great speech and was easily elected as "Sheriff Jackson" at Palmetto Boys' State.

Thus, began Robert's career as an activist. Dr. William "Bill" Hunter from Clemson, South Carolina, one of Robert's mentors and good friends, recalled:

Robert was a young man who looked even younger. He was
successful in his medical profession. He had a wonderful loving
family and nearly everything he touched turned to gold. I was
convinced that his star would reach a zenith that few men knew.
Robert was picked by organized medicine in South Carolina as a
leader. He was perhaps the youngest physician ever to chair the
Reference Committee of the South Carolina Medical Association,
which he did quite ably. He was picked as the first chairman of
the Standing Committee for Medical Specialties of the SCMA.
Additionally, he became one of the youngest directors of the South
Carolina Academy of Family Physicians.

One of Robert's classmates observed, "Robert accomplished
so much more than any of us; in hindsight, it was as if he knew
he had less time." I didn't believe that then and still don't. Robert
accomplished all that he did because he had a desire to live life at
its fullest — to act, to do, and to be. I can't help but smile and think
of a political phenomenon that Robert pulled in a US Senate race.
He had just begun to practice medicine in his early twenties, and
he wasn't particularly politically inclined. Nevertheless, he was
people-inclined, and the people of Clarendon County — black
and white, young and old, rich and poor, men and women — all
loved him.

It was about this time that a few of us around the state,
all political novices, thought that we could come up with an
outstanding candidate of outstanding character and elect him to
the US Senate. We persuaded W.D. "Bill" Workman, later editor
of *The State* newspaper, to oppose then incumbent Senator Olin
Johnston.

I asked Robert to be Clarendon County's chairman for
Workman's campaign, which he did in his usual energetic way.
While Workman came close to winning with a big Upstate vote,

he hardly carried a low-state county. I remember well the map of South Carolina covering the election. Other than Charleston in the Lowcountry, there was only one county shaded for Workman — Clarendon County. The night of the election, someone asked Bill Workman, "How did you carry Clarendon County?" He responded simply, "You ever heard of someone named Robert Jackson?"

Traditionally, all of the rural counties in South Carolina voted Democratic for many years. Robert used to laugh and say that he could hold the entire Republican County Convention in Clarendon at his kitchen table.

On another occasion, Robert ran for coroner in Clarendon County in June 1972. His older brother Jehu recalled, "He felt very strongly that the coroner should have some experience in medicine. He was convinced that many cases that were pronounced accidental were, in fact, intentional crimes."

Convinced that many suspicious deaths should be investigated, he was frustrated that he had no political influence over the coroner, a funeral home director with no medical expertise. Robert often appealed to the coroner, requesting an investigation of a death he considered suspicious. The coroner responded in a passive-aggressive fashion, "That would only cost the county unnecessary expenditures."

Deciding to take action, Robert ran for coroner but was defeated in this bid by the local funeral home director. His brother Jehu continued, "I heard a few folks comment that they were not going to vote for Robert because he was so busy in his medical practice and he was their doctor. They did not want him to have anything else to take him away from his practice of medicine." Others thought it was unfair for an affluent physician to take away the paid position of a funeral home director. The real issue that he was trying to address by running for office was being overlooked entirely!

Robert threw himself with his usual energy and enthusiasm into promoting the goals of the American Heart Association. South Carolina

was, and is, a perennial leader in strokes and heart attacks due to athero-
sclerotic vascular disease. Situated in what is commonly called the "stroke
belt," South Carolina also has the "fifteenth highest death rate from cardio-
vascular disease in the country." Robert lectured over the years on behalf
of the medical profession in an attempt to promote good heart health.
He spoke at churches and civic organizations teaching the importance of
proper diet, exercise, tobacco cessation, and medication compliance. Many
of the things that seem so common sense to us today were, in fact, strange
and alien to the rural populations of South Carolina in the 1960s and '70s.

Once again, Robert's oratorical skill and his knack for combining rural
country doctor stories about his heart patients (anonymously, of course)
with his quick wit delighted his audiences. The South Carolina Heart
Association repeatedly honored Robert for his passionate promotion of
heart health in rural South Carolina. Robert's sister-in-law, Katherine
Jackson, once remarked, "When Robert led a program, we all attended
because we didn't want to miss what he had to say. It was always very
interesting."

◆　◆　◆　◆　◆

"Son, if you want to be successful in life, just find a need and meet it.
Don't wait on anybody else. Don't depend on the government. Just take the
bull by the horns and meet that need yourself. If you have to organize other
people or an entire community, then do it. Success in business or ministry
depends on meeting needs that exist in the lives in the people around you."

Dad and I were driving home from his medical office. I had been
asking him questions about the sports medicine seminars he had started
and taught while I was in high school. He got pretty fired up talking about
it and ended with the above admonition. That mini-sermon has stood me
in good stead over the years. I understood clearly that I shouldn't grumble
or complain about unmet needs or wonder, "Why doesn't somebody do

something?" Dad taught me, "If it is to be, it is up to me."

"Dr. Jackson, the coach at Manning High School is on the line, asking if you will perform physicals on the football players once again this year."

Robert questioned, "Ask him how many?"

Still holding the phone, she promptly asked the coach how many physicals needed to be done, and then wide-eyed, she responded, "He said there would be fifty athletes."

Without hesitation, Dr. Jackson said, "Tell him I will be there."

His nurse hung up the phone, looked at him, and queried, "You're going to examine all fifty of them after you've seen sixty patients here in the office?"

He smiled at his nurse and replied quickly, "Not to worry. I'll just handle it."

Robert's interest in young people and their safety in the sports arena was exemplified by his willingness to examine so many athletes on a late afternoon after spending a full day at the office. He sincerely believed that if one could spot that potential hernia, hear that slight heart murmur, discover that unreported high blood pressure, or discover diminished vision, then corrective measures could be taken to ensure the young athlete's safety on the playing field. He advocated having trained medical technicians at all sporting events — particularly football games — and he personally attended every ball game possible. He often sat on the bench with the athletes in order to be instantly accessible in case of injury to a player. Most of the time, he was the only physician available for both teams, running back and forth to administer aid to either team needing medical help or advice.

I recall playing in a football game in tenth grade when an opposing team player's cleat struck me on the forehead, somehow entering between the face mask and top of the helmet. Unbeknownst to me, I sustained a laceration to the bridge of my nose and started bleeding vigorously. The blood and sweat mixed freely and quickly covered my entire face and jersey, but I was completely unaware. When back in the huddle, my good friend Bruce Hodge looked at me with wide eyes and exclaimed, "Dow Bo. You need to go to the sidelines." I looked down at my jersey, saw all the blood, still didn't know from where it came, and trudged off the field. As I took off my helmet, I saw Dad vault over the chain link fence and drop down to the field, which was several feet lower than the stands. In just a few steps, he had my head in his hands examining my wound. As the crowd gasped at the sight of all that blood, he merely said, "You'll be fine. It'll only take two stitches." And he was right. After the game, he placed two sutures and I was as good as new. All my teammates were amazed that my own dad sewed me up!

The coaching staff at Manning Christian Academy, where his children attended school, outfitted Dad with purple pants and a white shirt like those of the coaches. His family often accused him of forgetting his position as medical advisor in order to give unsolicited coaching advice to the coaches.

Robert's concern for student athletes was so intense that he organized a Sports Medicine Seminar to instruct coaches and trainers in the finer points of preventing injuries and heat strokes, but also the technique for treating those problems if they should occur. Robert's Sports Medicine Seminar was so popular that WIS-TV in Columbia, which provided television coverage for his first seminar, invited him to present a thirty-minute special in which he explained the main points of the program.

Robert strongly believed that a parent should attend every event in which his children were involved, whether it be a sporting contest, a concert, a play, or a beauty pageant. Unless he was out of town, Robert attended everything involving his own children. Abbot recalls, "Robert was such a vocal fan that I often had to find another seat on the bleachers out of earshot of his 'advice' to the referees."

He was convinced that an athlete or student should always give his very best. He was quite disappointed at the young man or woman who gave a half-hearted effort. "Robert approached sports as he did everything else

— with a 100 percent effort," recalls Abbot. "At the annual student-faculty basketball game, he would play so hard that I feared he might have a heart attack. It was not in him to signal for a substitute or admit he was not in adequate physical condition."

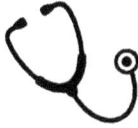

22

THE BIG SNOW

On February 9, 1973, the outside was cold and dreary with low-lying clouds. I left the school building to retrieve something from my car when snowflakes began to fall — not just any snowflakes, but giant goose feathers like I had never seen before. This was Manning, South Carolina — in the Deep South, to say we rarely had snow is an understatement, much less goose-feather snowflakes. Snow in our neck of the woods always generated excitement, but I tried to control the elation bubbling up in me as I walked back into the school building. I pretended nonchalance when I walked into my fifth period classroom and announced, "It's snowing outside," which was greeted with jeers and disbelief. Even so, half of the class ran to the windows and immediately began to "ooh" and "ah." It really was a beautiful sight. Snow in Manning, and in the middle of the day! Who would believe it? Usually, we would only get a dusting in the middle of the night (less than a half inch at the most) and by mid-morning it would be gone, hardly enough to make snowballs — such disappointment for little kids. However, this snow held real promise!

Much to our delight, school let out early — allowing us to get home, change clothes (although I don't remember any of us having proper clothes for snow), throw snowballs, and build snowmen before supper. Whoever heard of such a thing in our Deep South hometown? The snow just kept falling — thick and heavy — while the kids played in it with reckless abandon; the adults stood in their doors and windows, watching it fall in awe and amazement. Could this really be happening in our town? By supper time, eight inches of snow lay on the ground with no sign of letting up.

After supper, my mom set out candles in case the power went out. I was watching my dad read the newspaper as a fire roared in the fireplace (we rarely had occasion for such fires) when suddenly Dad sat straight up in his recliner, crumpled up the newspaper in alarm, and said out loud, "I-95." We all stared at him expectantly, and then he said, "If we can't travel on the roads in town, the people on I-95 can't travel either." Always decisive, he didn't hesitate. He first called his brother Ralph who lived twenty miles away in Gable, South Carolina, but whose house was only a few hundred yards off the interstate.

"Ralph, can you see I-95 from your house?"

"No, the snow's falling too thick."

"Well, go to the overpass, look both ways, then call me back and tell me what you see."

"Why?"

"Just go look and call me back. Hurry!"

We waited thirty anxious minutes before the phone rang.

"Doc, you won't believe it! There are cars and trucks backed up three or four cars wide as far as I can see in both directions. We gotta do something."

Immediately, my dad was on the phone calling the National Guard commanding officer in Manning to get out the troops. Carter Jones, the assistant fire chief in Clarendon County at the time, recalled in a personal interview, "Ceth Johnson, who was the commanding officer of the Army Guard in Manning; Homer Nash, the fire chief; and Dr. Jackson, the captain in the Air National Guard, assumed control in this crisis situation." It was obvious to me that the other men in leadership respected my dad's opinions, and they followed his guidance, as the following week would reveal. Dad next called McEntire Air National Guard base where he was stationed in Columbia, South Carolina, to ask for helicopter support; however, the cloud cover was so dense that the copters would be unavailable for three days, much to everyone's frustration. A few big trucks with big tires were still mobile, but the snow was already so deep that ordinary vehicles could not travel. Even tractor trailers were stranded on I-95. People on the interstate were beginning to run out of gas and in danger of freezing. Many people were more than fifteen-to-twenty miles from the nearest exit as long stretches of interstate existed between Orangeburg and Florence, South Carolina. This freak blizzard ultimately dumped twenty-four inches of snow between noon on Friday and 6:00 p.m. on Saturday. It became known as "The Big Snow of '73."

The Army Guard had several "deuce-and-a-half" vehicles that could travel in the deep snow, so they were soon mobilized and began to rescue people from the interstate. The rescued people were relocated to truck stops and motels, of which there was only one truck stop and two motels at the Manning exit on I-95. They were quickly overwhelmed with people. The sheer number of people coming in could not be handled by the Army Guard vehicles. Thankfully, Manning is an agricultural community filled with good-hearted people. The farmers in town were soon alerted to the impending disaster. By early Saturday morning, the bigger tractors available with forty-foot cotton trailers were easily plowing through the snow as if it were nothing going to the rescue of people they did not know. It was frightening and sobering to watch fifty to a hundred people at a time, wearing shorts and flip-flops, crying due to exposure, coming off the interstate standing in cotton trailers with metal mesh walls in freezing temperatures and howling winds. That picture of hundreds of miserable, nearly frozen people clutching the metal mesh walls of the cotton trailers is burned into my memory.

Carter Jones, the assistant fire marshal in Manning at the time, records in his book *A Legacy That Lives On*:

Had farmers and other citizens with heavy equipment not come to the aid of the tourists trapped on the interstate, many would have perished ... As the hours passed with no help in sight, hundreds of motorists trapped in their vehicles began to exit their vehicles and were seen scaling fences along the highways to trek their way to houses nearby seeking shelter and relief from the cold. Many a homeowner took in folks suffering from near hypothermia and provided hot soup, coffee, and a change of clothing. Many homeowners even allowed these destitute strangers to spend days and nights in their homes, and, as a result, lasting friendships were made, giving rise to the meaning of being a good neighbor.

All of my growing up years, there was a sign at the entrance to my hometown that read: "Manning, Known for Beauty and Hospitality." The events of the next week proved the veracity of that advertisement.

Sherry Stewart, a nursing student at USC in Columbia, South Carolina, at that time, recalls:

We stood in our backyard and watched the snow. We could not take our eyes off of it. We watched it so much, we could close our eyes and still see the flakes! We finally went to sleep only to wake up to a landscape we had never seen! ... The cold wind blew through us like knives. We, joined by some of our neighbors and friends, struggled against the snow and wind down to the end of our street where there was a guest house owned by the nearby motel. The guests had been stranded on I-95 just outside of town and were rescued by local farmers on tractors. The rescued, who were not from around here, came out of the guest house, inquired as to when the "road plows" would be clearing the roads, to which I laughingly replied, "There are no road plows or snow-clearing equipment. This is Summerton, South Carolina, in Clarendon County, South Carolina. It does not snow here!"

Sherry went on to become a nurse at Clarendon Memorial Hospital in Manning.

Soon, every church in town and the high school auditorium overflowed with people rescued from the interstate — people from every part of the eastern seaboard from New York to Miami, very few of whom were dressed for cold weather. Unfortunately, for those farthest from the exits, it took more than two days to rescue them. By that time, they were out of gas and freezing in their bitterly cold vehicles. As the churches ran out of spaces, many of our homes began to make room for those stranded. Our family welcomed a family from Gray Neck, New York, who stayed with us for nearly ten days until the roads thawed out enough to travel and to clear the tangled mess on the interstate.

I was a fascinated spectator to all of this winter wonderland, standing next to my dad, who helped coordinate much of the rescue and care of the people stranded in this blizzard. I traveled out on the interstate on a giant eight-wheel John Deere tractor, snug as a bug in a rug in the heated cab, to pick up people in their cars. We pulled a completely enclosed trailer, so people were happy to exit their cars and jump into our trailer, safe from the bitter wind. On one occasion, I flew in a helicopter with my dad out to a home where he went to deliver a baby at one house and sew up a laceration at another. As a seventeen-year-old with a brand-new private pilot's license, I was thrilled beyond words to fly in a military helicopter and see the winter wonderland from the air.

Carter Jones was stranded at a fire station in Sumter, South Carolina, until Monday morning — at which time a helicopter owned by Sharp Construction Company delivered him and hundreds of loaves of bread to the Clarendon County armory. Carter recalled, "We flew to general stores all over the county, dropping dozens of loaves of bread. We also dropped bread at remote homes with no access to the main roads. Later, we began to drop bales of hay from the helicopter to feed the farmers' cows since the snow had frozen solid for over one week."

ON LAUGHTER-SILVERED WINGS

Carter also wrote:

> There were other emergencies unfolding while the evacuations
> were taking place on the super slab (I-95). As shelters opened and
> thousands of people were flocking in, the issues of supplying these
> evacuees with food, cots, diapers, baby formula, blankets, and
> essential medications grew to crisis proportions. Grocery stores,
> pharmacies, and other merchants opened their doors to allow the
> shelters to take from their stocks until outside resources could be
> brought in to the impacted communities to provide additional
> relief.

I watched Dad and the Army Guard officers deliberate over important
decisions regarding food, blankets, and personnel distribution. I have to
say, even now, after all of these years, I was terribly proud of my father, his
demeanor, and his obvious leadership skills. In our interview, Carter said:

> The management of logistics and triage of the injured was
> referred to Dr. Jackson because of his natural leadership skills and
> his previous combat experience in chaotic situations in Southeast
> Asia. Dr. Jackson became the "go-to guy" for all health issues and
> injuries, of which there were many. When others were paralyzed
> by indecision and the enormity of the task, he always knew exactly
> what to do. He spent a lot of time traveling in the Army Guard
> deuce-and-a-half trucks traveling out into the county, caring for
> the injured and delivering babies.

Ed Fry, the hospital administrator at Clarendon Memorial Hospital
at that time, related to me that three days into the "Big Snow," it became
apparent that there were numerous guests at the local churches and the
National Guard Armory who were either drug abusers or who had been

taking prescription narcotics. These folks began to withdraw from their medications — whether illicit or prescribed, no one knew. According to Ed, these visitors began to create quite a disturbance at multiple locations around town as they began to experience withdrawal symptoms. About that time, a fist fight broke out at the high school auditorium, and someone vandalized Brunson's Pharmacy.

Ed related the following:

Robert came to me and said, "Ed, what are we going to do with all of these folks withdrawing from their medications? Some of them are becoming quite ill, and some are causing serious trouble."

"I don't know, Doc. What do you think?"

Obviously, Robert had thought about it, because he quickly responded, "I think we should write all of them a short supply of their medication and send them on their way as quickly as possible."

And that's exactly what he did, eliminating the riot that was brewing.

Thankfully, there were local pharmacies within walking distance of the churches and the armory where these prescriptions could be filled.

As a side note, I owned a 125-cc dirt bike that traveled easily in the deep snow, so I could get around when others could not. My friend Freddie and I found an old sheet metal Coke sign that was split in half. It made an awesome sled when towed behind the dirt bike. We found pristine, untouched snow in fields around town, and I pulled him in that sled like he was behind a motorboat. He slid on the untouched, frozen snow without any friction — "fast and furious." Haha!

At the end of ten days, the freezing temperatures abated, and the sun melted the ice-bound cars. All the stranded people who had no idea where their cars were located were loaded on school buses and driven down the interstate until they saw their cars. They were given five gallons of gas and directed to the nearest exit with a gas station. My mom corresponded with the family from Gray Neck for several years afterwards.

Carter Jones concludes his chapter entitled the "Snowstorm of 1973" with this observation: "In all of these stories, a common thread runs through each, depicting compassion of our states' citizens; sacrifice for strangers; great courage and bravery. Less than twenty people lost their lives as the result of the storm, most succumbing to exposure to the elements."

We all agree that twenty lives lost were far too many, but many thousands more were rescued up and down the I-95 corridor by the energy, creativity, and compassion of the citizens of Clarendon County and those adjacent. It has been forty-eight years since this historic, landmark event, but the people of my home county still share stories of the "Big Snow of '73."

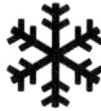

23

THE ENTERTAINER

Every doctor's medical bag is stuffed full of the interesting, the humorous, the heartbreaking, and the bizarre — such as the time Robert delivered triplets from a 400-pound patient in the bed of a small pickup truck in the hospital parking lot. She was too large to fit in the cab of a small truck and arrived too late to be transported into the hospital before the triplets arrived. He never tired of telling that story to his big city doctor friends with a minor amount of country doctor embellishment. However, not every physician can relate their experiences in a compelling fashion. Robert was the consummate storyteller and never reluctant to regale any audience with tales of his childhood, his family, or his medical patients (anonymously, of course).

According to Abbot, "Robert had perhaps the most unique sense of humor of any man I have ever known. He delighted in entertaining folks and was always the life of the party. Amusing stories (tall tales, if you will) flowed from his repertoire as easily as ordinary conversation. One never knew where reality ended and imagination began."

Robert and his immediate three older brothers — Carl, Scott, and Ralph — loved nothing more than to get together and take turns sharing the latest humorous anecdotes they had recently heard or personally experienced. They had a habit of writing the punch lines of their favorite stories on a scratch sheet of paper and sticking it in their wallets as a quick reminder. When they saw each other, they raced to see who could pull out their wallet first — like a quick-draw gunslinger contest — in order to share their latest and best anecdote. They started laughing at each other, however, before they ever got their wallets out — so much so that tears streamed down their cheeks. The brothers loved each other dearly, and they loved to share their stories with each other.

Dr. Larry Heavrin of Spartanburg, South Carolina, Robert's classmate in medical school, shared the following:

One of the tasks we were given as medical students in biochemistry class was to present a paper which was assigned to us by the doctor who was teaching the class, then head of the biochemistry department, Dr. McCord. Robert was assigned a paper which appeared in the *California State Journal of Medicine* and was written by Dr. Walter Alvary in 1916. The paper concerned the use of apocodeine, a new laxative with exceptional advantages. Robert presented his paper as probably no one else in the class would have been able to, giving not only the scientific portions in the paper, but adding some of his own humor. I still remember him telling about a man who was afflicted with chronic constipation who was from Tennessee, and when asked how he felt because of his longstanding constipation, he said, "Only a little distended." When this man was treated, Robert advised us that he was relieved of thirty-two gallons of feces, much to the delight and dismay of our class.

Robert frequently had stories to tell related to his growing up days in Manning [that he] connected to different subjects in the courses we were taking. At one time when we were talking about fungal infections and athlete's foot, Robert told about taking a corncob to scratch between his toes while in school. Some of our classmates stared in disbelief, while others laughed themselves silly.

We attended a meeting in Dallas, Texas, for an FAA seminar for aviation medical examiners. Robert was also in attendance, and during a presentation on air sickness, he was allowed to ask a question during which time he explained how it was possible to be airsick and still fly an airplane. He told of his experience when he was first learning to fly when he became violently ill, opened the window of his Piper Cub, stuck his head out, banked the plane over to the left so that he could vomit, and still maintained a fairly level flight plan. In the process of this, he had the entire audience in stitches — to the point that when the monitor for the seminar came to the platform following a presentation, he advised us that Robert would be given some time in the afternoon to tell some more stories. This was accomplished, and Robert entertained the crowd with his spontaneous humor for several minutes.

At the annual Fall Festival in Manning, Robert pulled together a costume complete with a mask and walked around at the local school carnival, never disclosing his identity until the costume contest, which he easily won several times. One year he was a farmer with overalls, straw hat, and pipe, carrying a stuffed mother pig with eight little pigs — attached at the appropriate places! Another time he was the Wookie Jedi, the furry giant from *Star Wars*, but wearing a gorilla mask and coveralls. On still another occasion, he was an old lady, complete with an old dress, purse, and old lady mask. He had a favorite old lady mask, which was so lifelike that one had to take a long look to determine that it was really a mask.

One time while wearing the old lady mask and covered with a sheet, groaning all the while, he had Kermit Holliday, his medical assistant, push him in a wheelchair through the waiting room of his office. Later, a patient commented to Kermit, "I know that patient was sick, but she was the ugliest old lady I ever saw." Robert got a lot of laughs retelling that incident.

Marie Mathis, a charge nurse at Clarendon Memorial Hospital,

remembers being called down to the emergency room to check a maternity
patient who was in labor:

I was posted on the second floor that night, and a fairly new
nurse was working the ER. When she called me, I promptly went
down to help her out. As I entered the ER, I could hear the moans
from behind the curtain of the patient I was to check. The ER nurse
gathered a glove and lubricant for me, and we went to the patient's
side to comfort her. The patient, with her brunette curls lying
against the pillow, had covered her face partially with the sheet and
was rubbing her stomach. I tried to reassure her as I was preparing
her for the exam when she threw back the sheet and threw a stuffed
animal at me and cried, "Oh, nurse, my baby has already come."
Well, the patient turned out to be none other than Dr. Jackson and
his Clemson orange-colored pig with little ones nursing, attached
to their mother. Of course, everyone really got a charge out of it.

Another time, he dressed himself like an old lady with a gray
wig, face mask, beads hanging over a well-proportioned bodice, a
shawl and handbag, and came strolling into the ER to check his
patients after the annual Halloween carnival. His patients got a really
big kick out of that. I had been told that he actually wore a mask of
Pluto, the Disney character with long, floppy ears, to a Clemson
football game. Can you imagine the other drivers' reactions?

Mrs. Mathis was correct. My family and I recall that old hound dog
mask quite well, as Dad pulled it out many times while we rode down
the highway. Reactions were priceless. We children laughed with childish
abandon seeing the consternation on the surprised faces of people in
adjacent vehicles when they glanced over and caught a glimpse of our
dad in that mask. Drivers and passengers punched each other to get the
other's attention, then pointed at him. The snout on that mask was about

two-and-a-half feet long, so he had to keep the side window open in order to accommodate the mask when he turned and looked at people in cars beside him. Our mother looked on with terrible chagrin, but we children loved the entertainment.

A favorite story was the time he dressed in overalls, flannel shirt, straw hat, moustache, and corncob pipe, and flew his airplane to Hilton Head Island for the South Carolina Family Physician's annual meeting. He received many strange looks at the airport and in the taxi to the hotel, but the most quizzical looks came from his fellow physicians with whom he mingled and conversed. Finally, he walked up to his good friends, Bill Hunter and Marion Dwight, who recognized his voice and one exploded, "Damn you, Robert Jackson. Nobody in the world would do this but you!"

On another occasion, Robert and Abbot went on a Caribbean cruise with some of their friends, during which they attended an evening enter-tainment show. During the intermission, the musicians lingered a little long and the crowd became restless. Perceiving this, Robert jumped up on the stage, grabbed the microphone, and began to tell his homespun country doctor stories, much to the delight of the assembled crowd. The crowd held their sides and cried with laughter. When the musicians returned, the crowd booed them off the stage and begged Robert to continue telling his stories. He was more than glad to comply, for he was then in his element.

Robert loved to entertain so much that social events at his home and his lake house on Lake Marion were common events. He enjoyed inviting the neighbors over to churn ice cream on hot summer evenings. He hosted his medical staff with cookouts, and most of all he enjoyed inviting his older siblings over for hamburgers on the grill or a pig-picking. At the family events, the younger brothers almost always competed for center stage in their storytelling and their remembrance of their childhood adventures. None had as much good fodder or humor as Robert did when he shared the happenings of his medical practice.

He loved to tell about when his eighteen-year-old part-time receptionist,

Peggy Sue Richburg, was instructed to enter into the ledger charges for a circumcision he had performed earlier that day in the hospital. She responded naïvely by saying, "Oh, was it a boy or a girl?" Robert said a brief anatomy lesson had to follow.

Anna Lynn Floyd, a first cousin who also worked at the office, enjoyed hearing Uncle Robert tell this story:

One day a gentleman came in, and the receptionist, Peggy Sue Richburg, whose voice carried really well, asked him his name. He told her that his name was Hardy Herring, at which point she asked him again a little louder, "What's your name?" He responded again, "Hardy Herring." By this time, they had the full attention of everyone in the waiting room. Peggy Sue, even more loudly, said, "I know you are hard of hearing, but — what — is — your — name?" He again very patiently said, "My name is Hardy Herring." Everyone in the reception area nearly fell into the floor laughing. Ever after that day, Uncle Robert could mention this to any one of us working that day, and the laughter started all over again.

Dr. Bobby Ridgeway relates a story that Robert shared with the EMTs at the ER late one night. The story goes like this in Robert's words:

One of my [Robert's] senior citizen patients groaned and complained loudly in the waiting room as she waited to be seen. She suffered from rather severe arthritis in both knees and required a wheelchair. Her groaning disturbed the entire waiting room and her family who was with her. At last, her time came to be seen. I injected both knees with cortisone and lidocaine, waited thirty minutes, then rechecked her. The beneficial effect was rather miraculous! Her pain had mostly resolved, and she was standing unassisted. After seeing her standing unassisted, an idea popped in my head. I pushed her in the wheelchair into the waiting room and commanded her in a loud voice, "Stand up and walk," which she promptly did, to the amazement of the entire waiting room. Dad finished by saying, "I'm here to tell you that a revival nearly broke out in that waiting room."

Robert also loved to organize travel trips to Clemson football games, especially end-of-season bowl games. In 1977, Clemson played in the Gator Bowl in Jacksonville — the game that ended in infamy for Ohio State Coach Woody Hayes when he punched Clemson player Charlie Baughman, thus effectively ending his coaching career. Sitting in the end zone beside my brother Richard when the incident occurred, I looked at Richard and exclaimed, "That coach just hit our player!"

Richard responded, "He sure did!" We stared at each other wide-eyed as the mêlée on the field continued.

Robert organized the bus trip to this game. Calling himself the "Jackson Travel Agency," he busily made motel and meal arrangements, chartered the bus, sent out newsletters, and arranged tickets. He was a self-appointed host and entertainer for the trip. He regaled the bus passengers with his tall tales and finally gave free blood pressure checks to anyone willing to endure the comments, such as, "Are you sure you're still alive?" and "Boy! I bet your wife has a hard time getting your pressure up!" However, the funniest act was when he dipped into his medical bag, pulled on a plastic glove, and walked down the aisle, shouting, "Next!" That ended the free medical checkups!

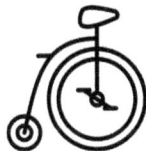

24

PEAS IN A POD

All of our growing up years, my brothers and I heard people in our hometown say to us, "You are Dr. Jackson's boys, aren't you?" This was a good stimulus for good behavior. Everywhere we went, folks looked at us, cocked their heads to one side, and said, "You belong to Dr. Jackson, don't you?" Any misconduct got back to him in a skinny minute. I guess it was a combination of our physical appearance and our distinct way of speaking.

My brother Richard sat on the porch of a clubhouse in Myrtle Beach, waiting for a golf tournament to begin, drinking iced tea, and talking to a stranger. The gentleman looked at him, cocked his head and said, "You know, you remind me of a good friend of mine from Manning. Did you know Dr. Robert Jackson?"

Richard laughed out loud and replied, "Well, as a matter-of-fact, I do. He was my dad."

They both laughed then. When Richard told me this, I told him, "It's the voice, Richard, it's the voice. We all sound just like our dad. We are all peas in a pod."

My daughter was once employed in a photography studio in Louisville, Kentucky. A customer looked at her and said, "You're Dr. Robert Jackson's daughter, aren't you?"

Stunned, she answered, "My father is in Spartanburg, South Carolina, and I'm here. How did you connect us that far apart?"

The female customer replied, "I worked with your father in Labor and Delivery at Mary Black Hospital in Spartanburg for years. You look just like him, and you sound just like him. I would recognize one of his children anywhere."

In amazement, Hannah called immediately to tell me about this encounter, to which I replied, "Precious, you better not ever get into any trouble in Louisville, because I will know about it before the sun goes down."

Laughing out loud, she exclaimed, "You are right, Dad, you are so right!"

My sister, Anne, and I knew at an early age that we wanted to go into the medical field like our father. She graduated with a biology degree, and I ended up as a family medicine doctor just like Dad. One of my younger brothers is now a pharmaceutical rep. I recall my father teaching me the anatomy of the heart and the cardiopulmonary circulation using a large over-sized model of the heart when I was in the sixth grade, which I promptly explained to my science class at school. My teacher, who also taught the twelfth-grade science class, took me straight from my class to her twelfth-grade class and had me repeat the lesson for them. I thought nothing of it, but I recall the amazement on the faces of the twelfth-grade boys who were struggling to master the cardiopulmonary circulation. They were amazed to hear a sixth-grade punk explaining it to them. The amazement turned to disgust, and I don't think the lesson went over all that well. Nevertheless, I loved medical science at an early age and knew that I would follow in my father's footsteps. When folks asked me if I was going to be a doctor when I grew up, I always emphatically answered, "Yes!"

When I was in college, I participated in a Christian college ministry group. If I ever shared with the group an insight from my Bible studies or taught a Bible lesson, I often heard fellow students say, "Robert, that was so encouraging." I heard it so often that it baffled me — until some years later, I heard a pastor teach a lesson on spiritual gifts, and I began to understand that my spiritual giftedness was exhortation/encouragement. I have opportunities to do plenty of Bible teaching, and some suppose that "teaching" is my spiritual gift — but even when I teach, the primary impact is encouragement. The listeners go away encouraged to obey the Lord or walk in righteousness.

I share this because I am confident that Dad's spiritual gift was exhortation as well. He had superlative oratorical skills, with many opportunities to speak in front of varied audiences. My impression was that the primary impact was encouragement — usually to action or participation in a cause that he was representing, whether it was the American Heart Association, the rescue squad, or remembering the prisoners of war (POWs). He and I are alike in that regard — peas in a pod.

Over the years, he was an encourager to many family and friends on a personal level. Asa Hatfield said that when he first opened his pharmacy in Manning, business was really slow and:

> Dr. Jackson often stopped by just to ask how things were going. I told him business was slow. He bucked me up and told me to "Hang in there. Things will get better." Patients came in with a prescription and asked for Dr. Jackson's nephew, the pharmacist. I knew then that he had sent them to my store. He had told them that I was his nephew since I was married to his niece, Angie. He was such an encouragement to me in those early days. Whenever he left my store, he had me feeling like the store was a big success and everything was great. He was a great morale builder for me, and I'm sure he was for his patients as well.

Mac Davis, a retired Spartanburg physician and medical school classmate of Dad's, called me and said, "I heard you were writing a book about your dad. Well, I would like to contribute a couple of stories, if I may." I replied instantly, "Of course, I always love hearing stories about Dad."

Dr. Davis continued:

I worked at the Manning hospital the summer after your
father worked there. I believe he was an intern at the time, and
I was a rising senior medical student. He gave me a ride from
Charleston to Manning, and all the way there I fretted that I would
do something foolish that would injure a patient. Robert was such
an encouragement to me, telling me repeatedly that I would do
fine, to just remember my training. I really needed his words.
He provided just the boost I needed. When I got to Manning, I
assisted my brother, Dr. Marion Davis, in a surgical procedure.
The OR nurses told me that the summer before, during one of the
surgeries when the surgery was completed, the sponge count was
off by one sponge. They counted and then recounted. They were
still off by one sponge. The nurses were in a big fizz. Just as my
brother, Dr. Davis, was about to explore the abdomen looking for
the lost sponge, Robert lifted his foot and there was the missing
sponge. He had been intentionally standing on it the whole time.
He and Dr. Davis got a big laugh out of it, but the nurses frowned
at the both of them.

When it came to our college studies, Dad warned my sister and me
not to cram right before an exam. He challenged us to study all of our class
notes and reading assignments every day from one exam to the next, so
we were always caught up and never needed to "cram" the night before an
exam. That advice served us well all the way through college and, for me,
through medical school. I often had little to do the night before exams
in college because I had studied my notes all along and knew them by
heart. Medical school, of course, was different because of the volume of
reading required. Nevertheless, his encouragement to stay "caught up" was
invaluable. He always said, "Never put off until tomorrow what you can do

today." The advice he told us about college study habits was not just for us kids. He strongly supported Mom in her desire to complete her studies as well. A few years after they returned to Manning and set up the medical practice, Mom began taking college courses. I recall her studying late at night while coordinating the activities of a busy family, including helping us with all of our homework. Oh, my! In spite of the busyness of her life, she graduated from Francis Marion College. No one was prouder than our dad, the encourager.

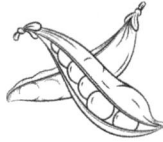

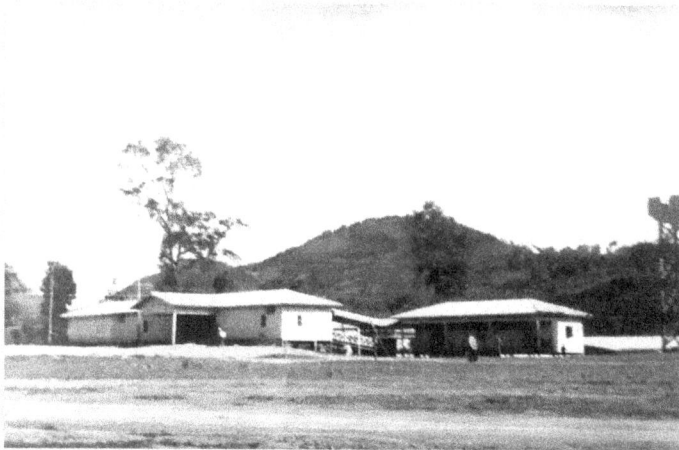

Chapter 15 —
San Sook
Hospital at
Sam Thong

Chapter 15 —
Hospital ward

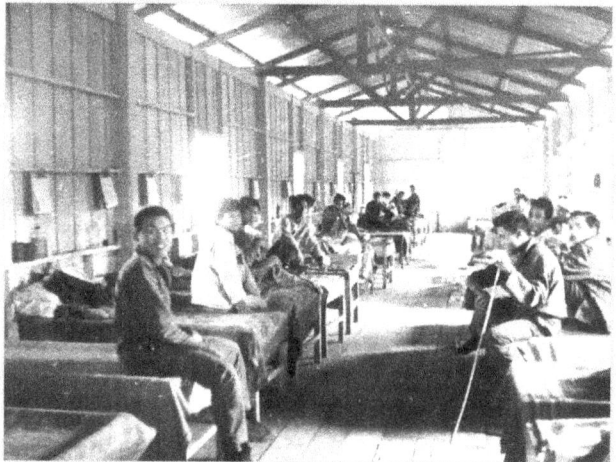

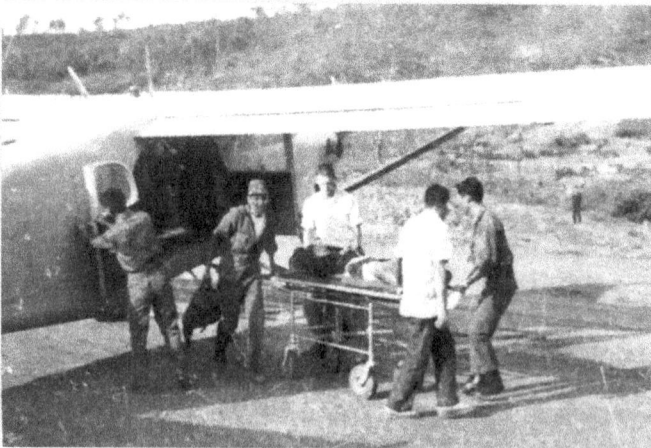

Chapter 15 —
Offloading
wounded
from plane

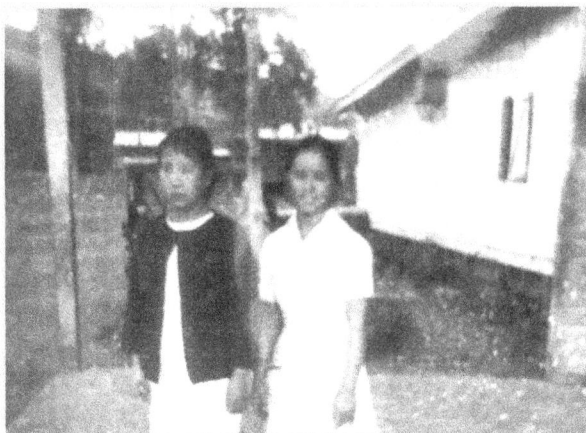

Chapter 15 —
Laotian nurses

Chapter 15 —
Captain Jackson
(left) and Dr.
Khammoung
(right)

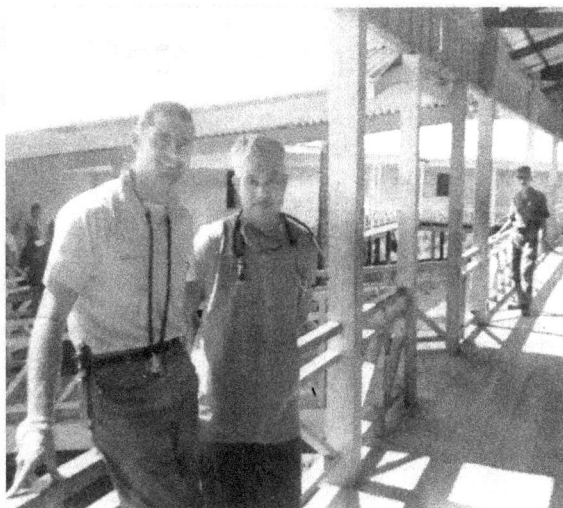

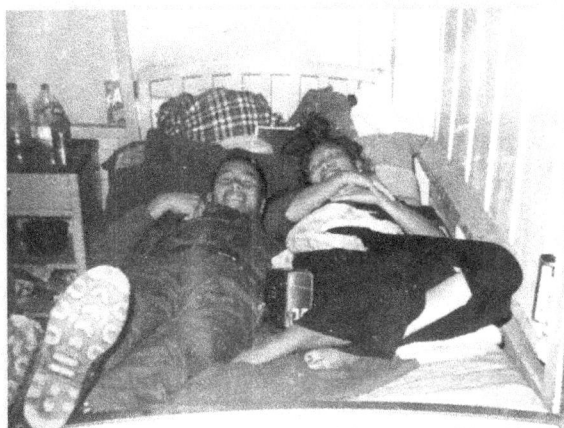

Chapter 15 —
Patient's family

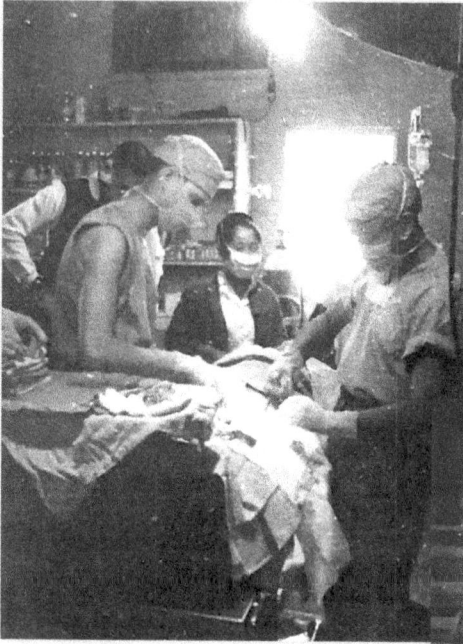

Chapter 15 —
Captain Jackson in OR

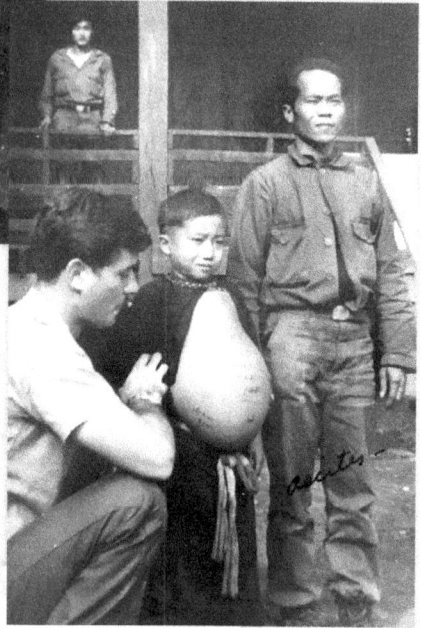

Chapter 15 — Child with malaria and
with ascites secondary to malnutrition

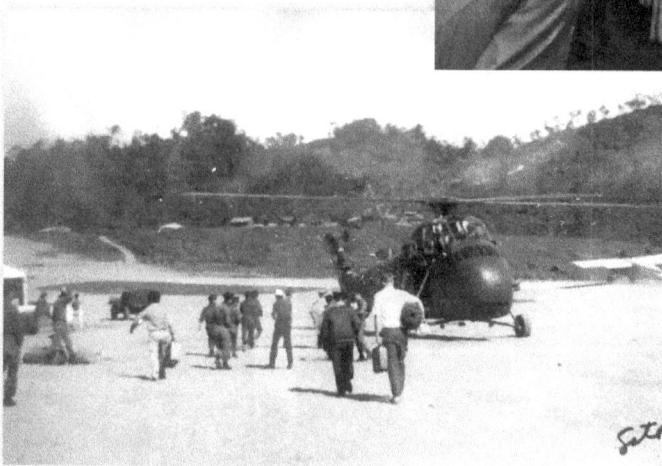

Chapter 15 —
Captain
Jackson
traveling
to outlying
village via
helicopter

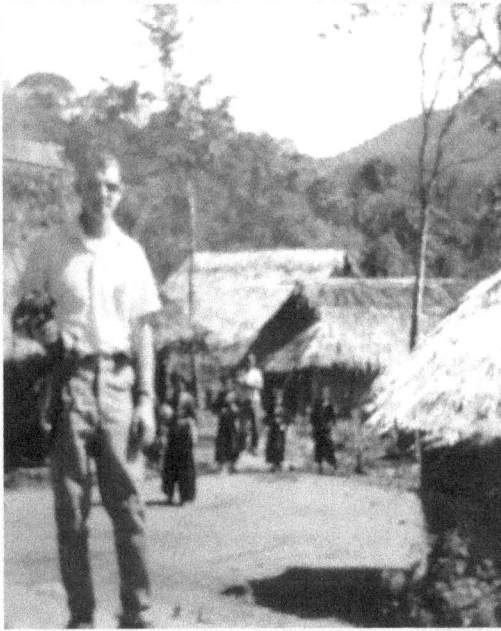

Chapter 15 —
Captain Jackson visiting
Hmong village

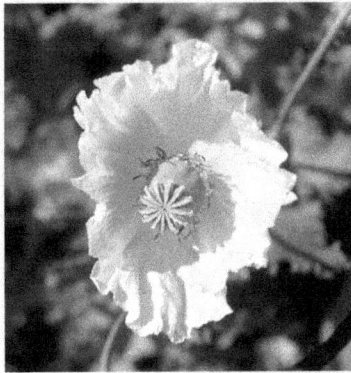

Chapter 15 — Poppy flower
important to Hmong economy

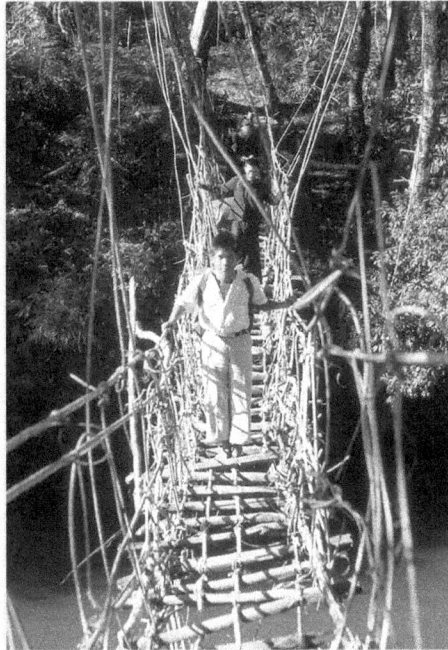

Chapter 16 —
Typical Southeast Asian log bridge

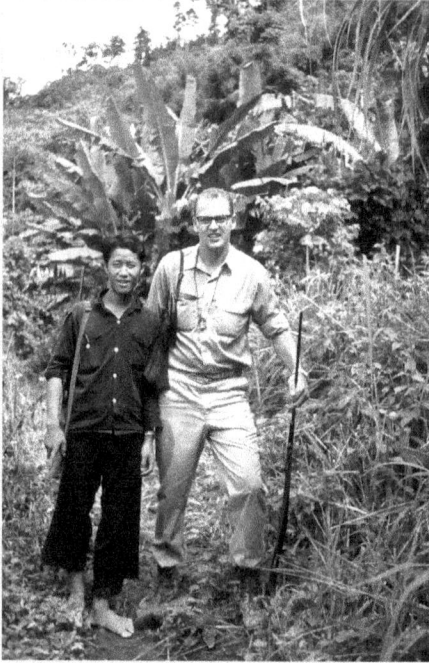

Chapter 16 —
Pastor Don Scott

Chapter 18 —
Flight Surgeon
of the Year, 1966

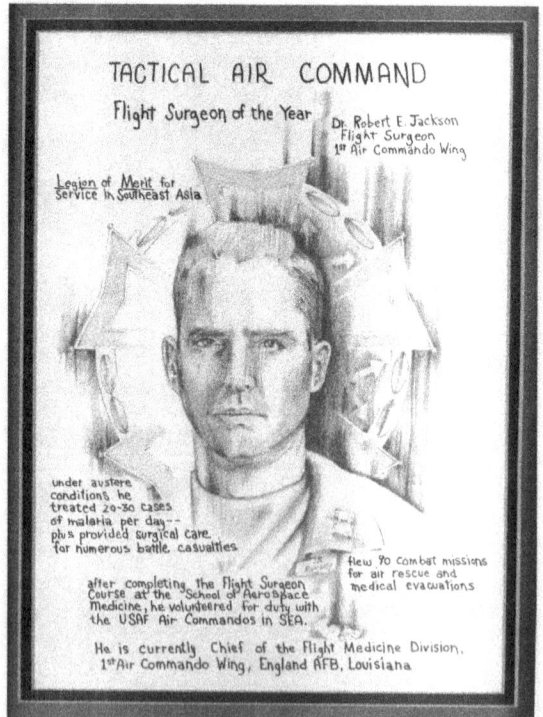

TACTICAL AIR COMMAND

Flight Surgeon of the Year

Dr. Robert E. Jackson
Flight Surgeon
1st Air Commando Wing

Legion of Merit for
Service in Southeast Asia

under austere
conditions he
treated 20-30 cases
of malaria per day--
plus provided surgical care
for numerous battle casualties

flew 90 combat missions
for air rescue and
medical evacuations

after completing the Flight Surgeon
Course at the School of Aerospace
Medicine, he volunteered for duty with
the USAF Air Commandos in SEA.

He is currently Chief of the Flight Medicine Division,
1st Air Commando Wing, England AFB, Louisiana

Highlights of Clarendon Week of Concern

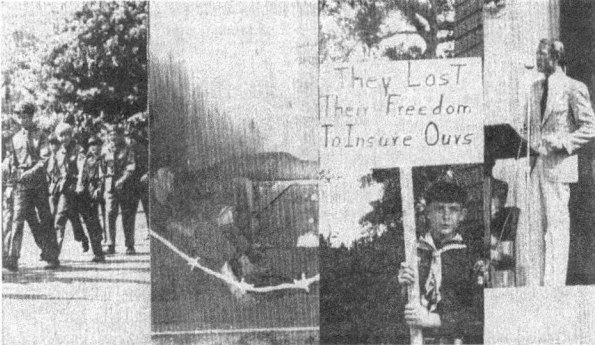

*Chapter 19 —
Week of Concern
activities: John Reed,
holding sign; guest
speaker Rep. Floyd
Spence (far right)*

Left to right, respectors carry the American colors in the parade; combatants not committed. Boy Scouts from Troop 301. Floyd Spence speaks to the assembled crowd. (Photos by Bruce Johnson)

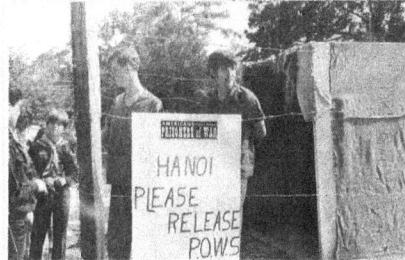

*Chapter 19 — "Robin" (left)
and friend Larry McCord
(right) in mock POW camp*

Acting POW's

Manning High School sophomores Robin Jackson and Larry McCord dramatized the condition of POW's in a stockade on the court house grounds. (Photo by King)

Parade Ends Concern Week

Climax of the Week of Concern in Manning for POW-MIA's was a parade Friday with the theme of patriotism.

Following the parade through town, special ceremonies were observed at the court house.

Guest speaker for the POW rally was Congressman Floyd Spence, R-SC, active in the Naval Reserve in the Columbia area and now serving on the U. S. Armed Services Committee.

Rep. Spence charged that American POW's are being used as "pawns" by the Communists. He added that he had joined with other congressmen in proposing the release of all POW's on both sides to a neutral country.

"The President made just such an offer, and Sweden offered to receive the prisoners; but Hanoi declined the proposal," Spence said.

In his talk Spence described some of the tactics used by the Communists to demoralize the men and their families and told of an interview he had with an American Navy lieutenant about the Communist brainwashing methods.

"This man was allowed to read only certain writings of Dr. Spock, selected portions of the Congressional Record, speeches by leading 'doves', and the 'Washington Post.'

"If anyone still doubts that 'peaceniks' in this country are playing into the hands of our enemy, this should convince them," Spence added.

Spence was introduced by Joseph O. Rogers, Manning attorney.

Special guests at the rally were wives of POW's residing at Shaw Air Force Base. They were Mrs. Hershel Morgan, Mrs. Marvin Lindsey, Mrs. Robert Stubberfield and Mrs. Bobby Ray Bagley.

Part of the week's activities included the erection of a replica of North Vietnam prisoner stockades on the court house grounds. Robin Jackson and Larry McCord, Manning High School sophomores, played the part of prisoners to dramatize the condition of U. S. prison-

Overall chairman for the week in Clarendon County was Dr. Robert Jackson. During the week Dr. Jackson spoke in the schools where petitions were signed to be delivered to North Vietnamese officials at Paris Peace Talks by Mrs. John C. West. Petitions were also signed in churches.

A proclamation for observance of the week had been issued by Manning Mayor Pansy Ridgeway. She requested all merchants to fly flags.

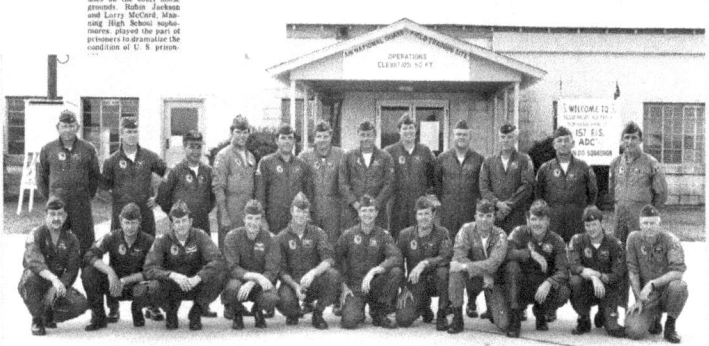

*Chapter 19 — Two-week summer camp in Savannah, 1973, with Air
National Guard unit, pilots and medical staff; Robert (front and center)*

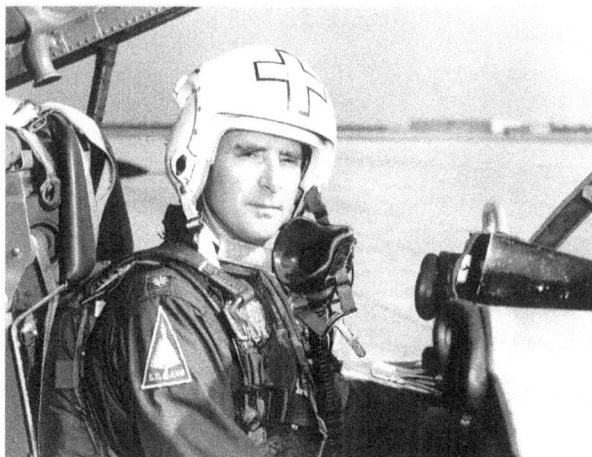

Chapter 19 —
Flight surgeon in
F-102

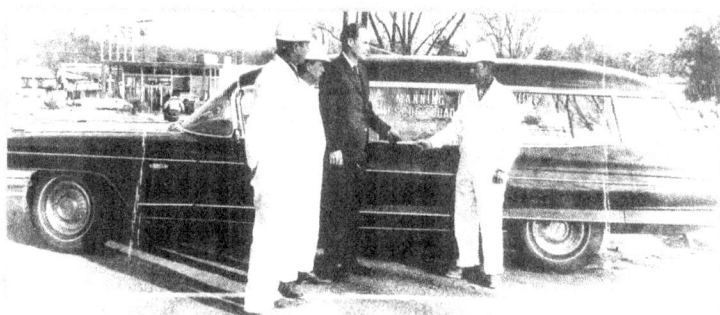

Chapter 20 — Original rescue squad vehicle. Left to right: Homer Nash,
Jerry Lea, Howard Elkins, J.D. Daniels (photo courtesy of Carter Jones)

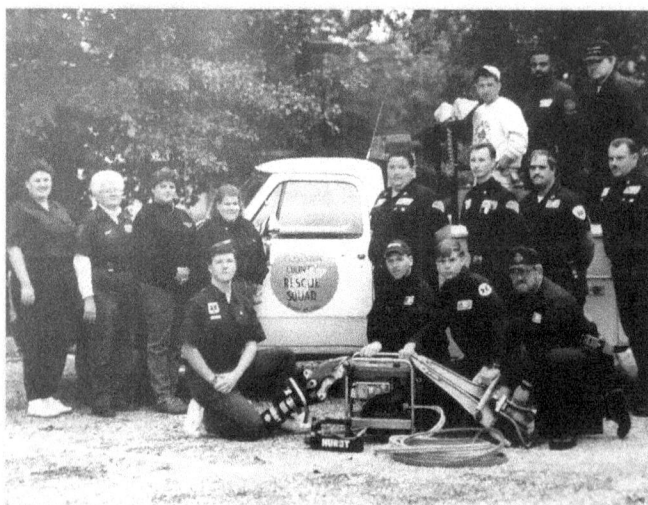

Chapter 20 —
Clarendon
County rescue
squad (photo
courtesy of
Carter Jones)

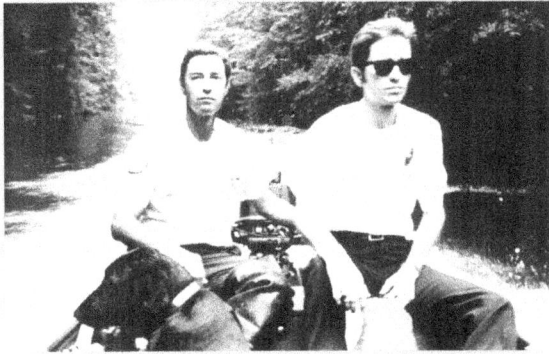

Chapter 20 —
J.D. Daniels (left) and
Carter Jones (right),
during flood of June
1973 (photo courtesy
of Carter Jones)

Chapter 21
— Citizen
statesman
in training
at Palmetto
Boys' State
— Robert,
first on left,
bottom row

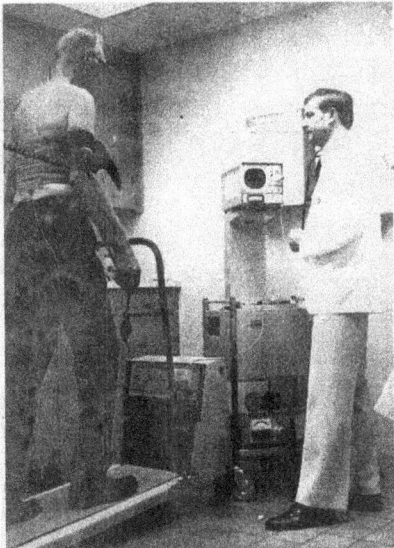

PAGE 2-B   The State: South Carolina's Largest Newspaper   COLUMBIA, S. C., WEDN

June 17, 1953 'Sumter County' Officers at Boys' State

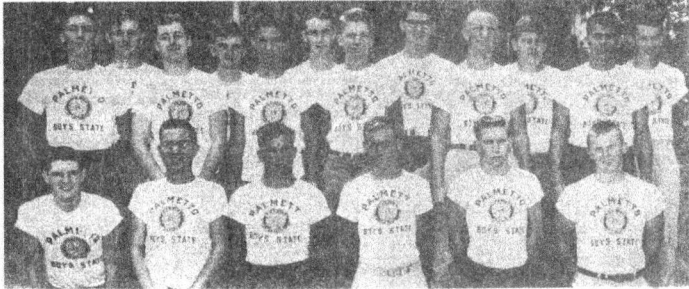

The picture above shows the Boys' Staters elected to offices of the mock county of Sumter. First row, left to right: Sheriff, Robert Jackson; senator, Lawton Salley; coroner, Dennis Caddel; clerk of court, Homer Jones, attorney, Gene Kelly, and representative, John Brooks. Second row, left to right: Senator, Robert Wall; representative, Boodle Hall; circuit Judge, Billy Sonenshine; representative George Bohlen; senators, Bob Johnston and Johnny Oliver. Back row, left to right: Representative, William Sealy; representative, Park er Dunlap; superintendent of education, Hal Anderson; representative, Eddie Strong; county treasurer, Tom Haskell, and representative Hugh Hawkins.

Chapter 21 —
Avant-garde stress testing in
1970s; one of his first stress test
patients — his brother Billy

DR. ROBERT JACKSON of Manning gives a patient a stress test. The equipment and testing technique were recently featured in a national medical magazine for family practitioners. In the article, Dr. Jackson advises medical colleagues to use the test regularly in their general practice to help diagnose "silent heart disease."
(Medical News Photo)

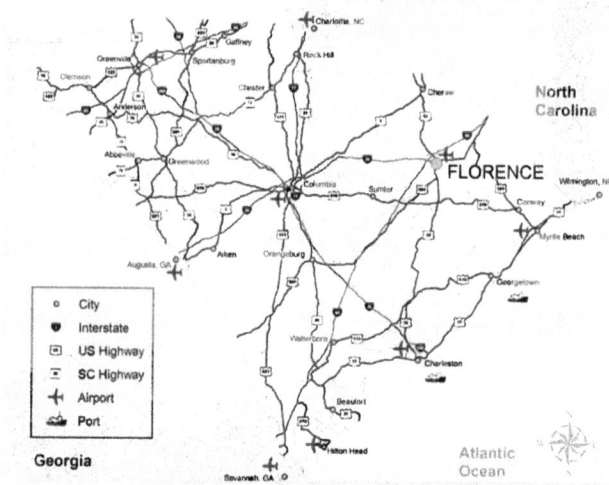

*Chapter 22 —
South Carolina
road map showing
ninety-mile stretch
of interstate
paralyzed from
"1973 blizzard,"
from Florence to
Orangeburg*

*Chapter 22 —
Summerton,
South
Carolina, ten
miles from
Manning*

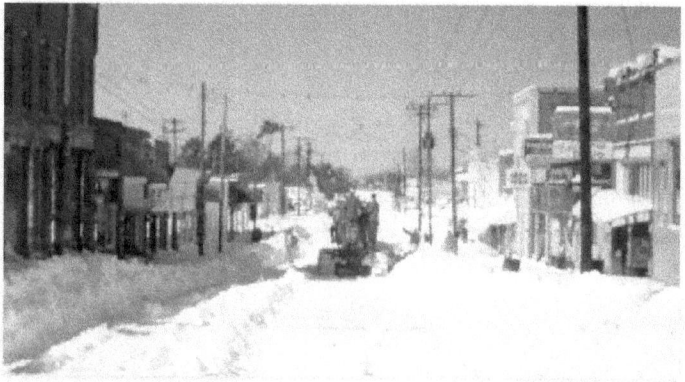

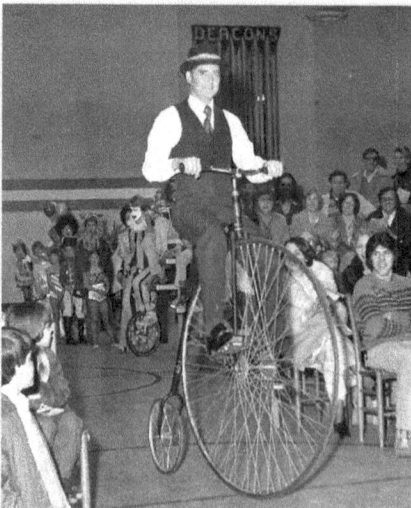

*Chapter 23 —
Robert at fall festival*

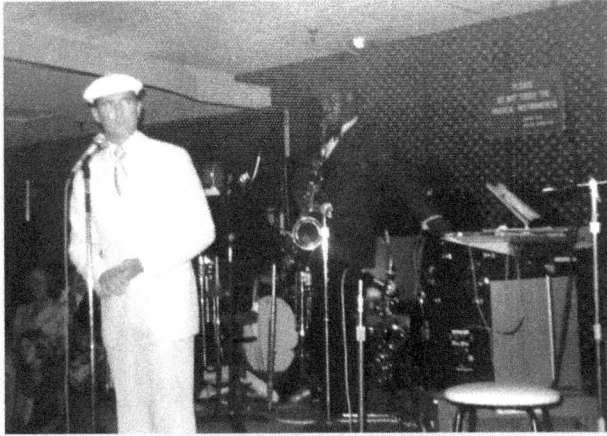

Chapter 23 —
Robert telling
country doctor
stories on the
cruise ship

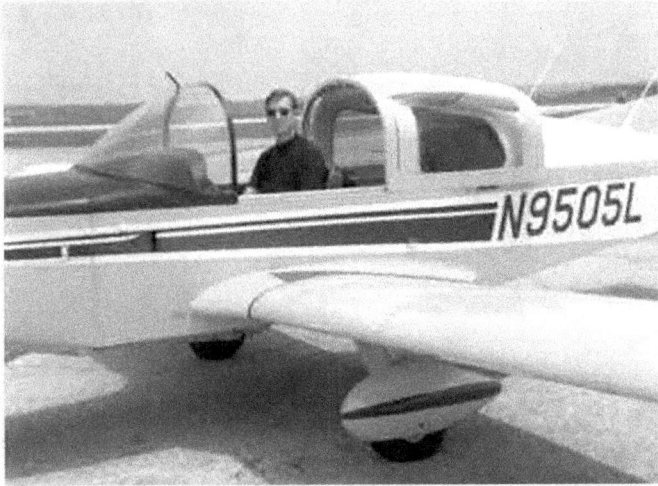

Chapter 26 —
Grumann
American
Traveler, Dad's
first plane

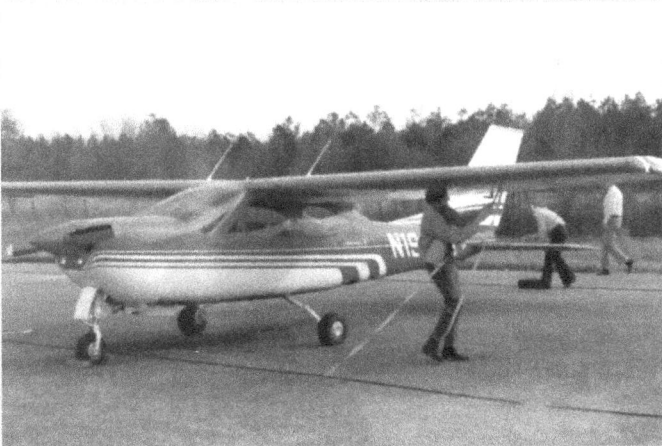

Chapter 26 —
Cardinal RG,
Dad's second
plane

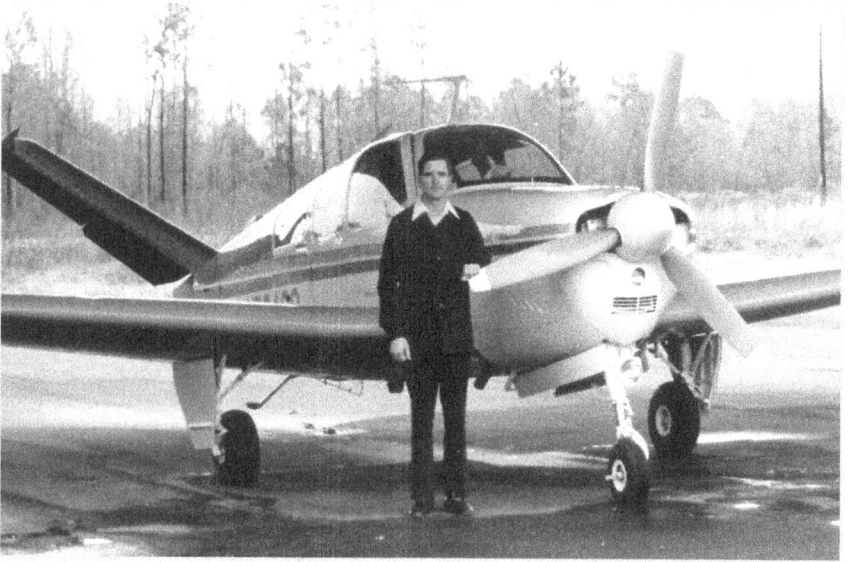

Chapter 26 — Beechcraft Bonanza, Dad's dream plane

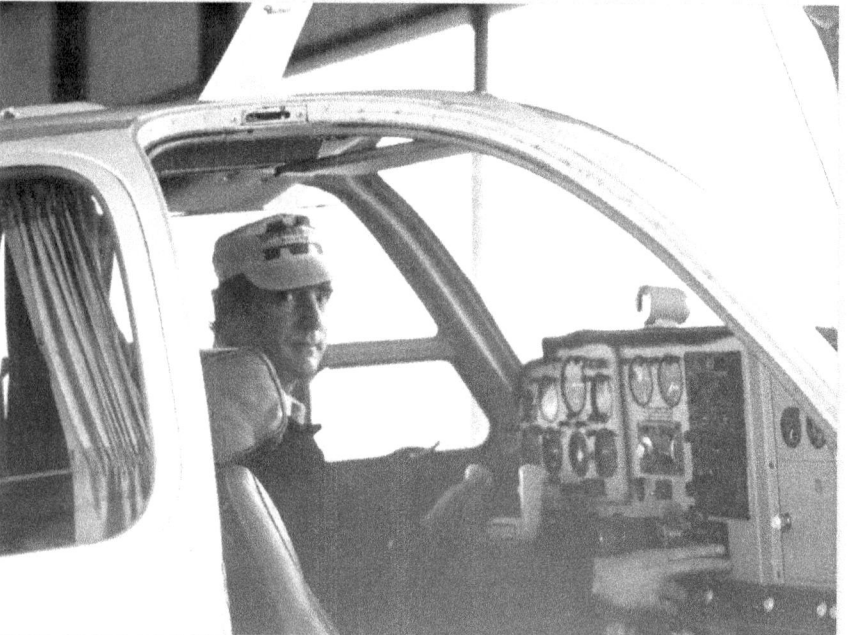

Chapter 26 — Dr. Jackson wearing painter's hat

The Painter's Hat Is The Needed Assurance

Mac McLeod

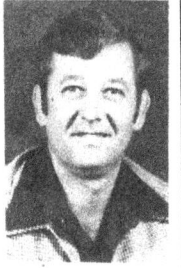

ITEM
SPORTS EDITOR

Chapter 26 —
"Faith and Trust" — part
of "The Painter's Hat Is the
Needed Assurance," written by
Mac McLeod with The Sumter
Daily Item, December 11, 1975

Faith And Trust

Everyday we place our trust in the hands of someone or something, whether it be in sincereness of someone indicating a turn at an intersection or our car getting us safely to work. Trust in others is a part of life.

But perhaps never do we place so much faith in another individual as we do in an airplane pilot. Once you buckle up in a plane seat, you are at the total mercy of the ability of that one man to take you from the ground into the heavens and bring you back down in one, breathing piece.

It's a big responsibility and although there are many who take to the airways, there are also only a small minority who are totally capable.

DOCTOR ROBERT JACKSON IS A MEMBER of that small group.

Back when I was an aviation storekeeper in the Navy, I would fly in anything. It was an adventure, something that broke the monotony of everyday service life. Flights on and off an aircraft carrier were the most exciting things around and I didn't miss many opportunities.

But the closer I got to getting my discharge, the less I enjoyed flying. As we used to say, "I was getting too short to be taking chances".

My flight from Seattle, Wash. to my home following my release was to have been my last. I swore up and down if I could make it one more time I wouldn't get back in one of those things.

And I kept my promise to myself for quite some time. Then one day I had the chance to go up in a light plane and took it and it was

Continued On Page 4B

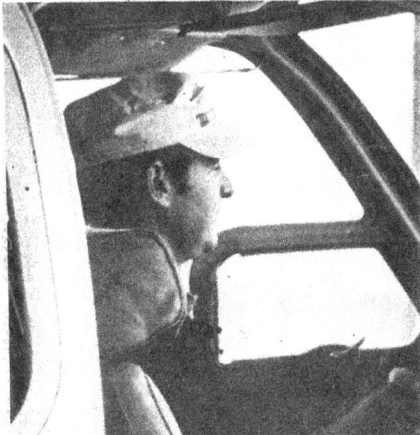

The Sumter Daily Item

VOL. 83   No. 282   Founded Oct. 15, 1894   Sumter, S.C., Tuesday Afternoon, September 12, 1978

Search For Manning Doctor
Continues On Land

Manning Doctor Feared Downed

ALEXANDRIA, La. (AP) — Rescue planes were searching today for a single-engine aircraft possibly carrying a South Carolina physician which winked off radar screens after hitting a storm.

The family of Dr. Robert Jackson of Manning, said he disappeared Sunday while flying to Houston.

Civil Air Patrol planes and a state police helicopter were scouring the area between here and Woodworth for a Beechcraft Bonanza which may either have crashed or made an emergency landing, a CAP spokesmen said.

The spokesman said the pilot was in contact with a radar center in Houston when he radioed that he had encountered turbulence at 8,000 feet 8 miles southwest of England Air Force Base.

The plane, which had been flying from Hattiesburg, Miss. to Houston, disappeared from the radar minutes later at 2:41 p.m. Sunday.

Manning Pilot Missing

ALEXANDRIA, La. (AP) —
~~~ ~ ~~~~ ~~~~~~~~ and

Plane Missing   The State

Search Continues For S.C. Surgeon

ALEXANDRIA, La. (AP) — Seven airplanes and an estimated 70 people on the ground searched wet forestland southwest of here Tuesday for a South Carolina pilot who disappeared on a flight to Houston.

Lt. Col. Les Hopper of the Civil Air Patrol in New Orleans said five fixed-wing aircraft and two helicopters were encountering "satisfactory" though marginal" flying conditions after the weather cleared enough to permit an air search to continue.

Jackson, a Vietnam veteran, was rated an excellent pilot by those who knew him, a CAP spokesman said.

Meanwhile, Manning Mayor Pansy Ridgeway said the disappearance of Dr. Jackson's plane has "saddened and shocked" the town.

Mayor Ridgeway said the entire town is "anxiously awaiting" the hopefully good news concerning him. Should it be bad news, Manning will suffer a great loss. He did have a family practice here and he was very

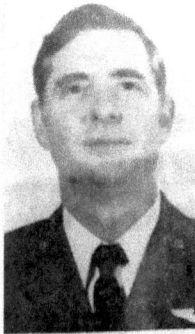

DR. ROBERT L. JACKSON

The State — Tuesday, Sept. 12

Manning Doctor's Plane Disappears During Mississippi To Texas Flight

From Staff And Wire Reports

ALEXANDRIA, La. — Fixed-wing
aircraft and helicopters searched which

Chase said seven fixed-wing aircraft and four helicopters, two from the sheriff's office and state police,
and two from Fort Polk, joined the

and a 1961 graduate of the Medical College (now University) of South Carolina.

He was the Legion of Merit a

The Manning Times

First Of All: The News of Clarendon County Completely And Accurately Reported

Manning, South Carolina Wednesday, September 20 1978   15 CENTS PER COPY

On Flight To Houston
Dr. Jackson Dies In Plane Crash

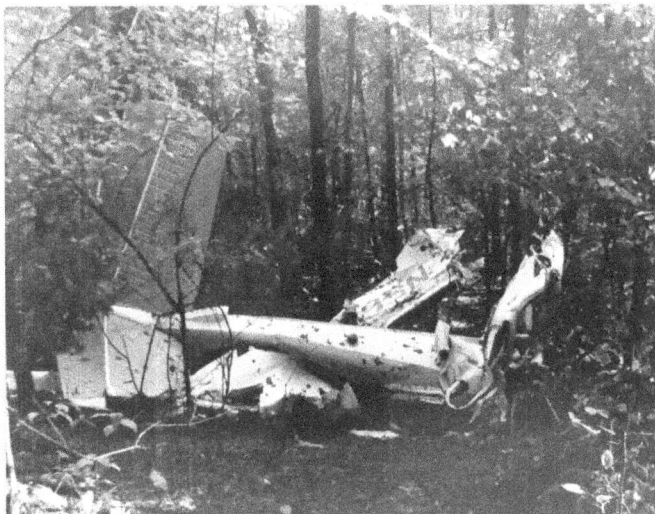

Chapter 28 — Scene of accident

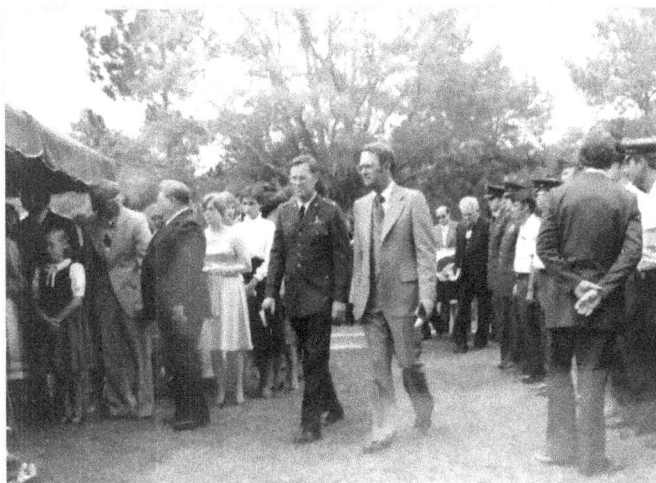

Chapter 28 — Dr. Sullivan and Chaplain Jerry Hammett

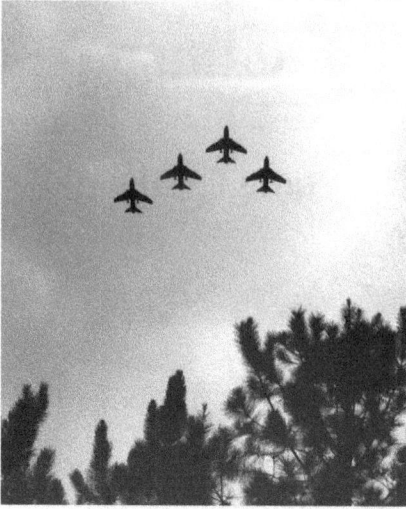

Chapter 28 — McEntire Air National Guard jets fly over

Chapter 28 — Local pilots fly over in "missing man" formation

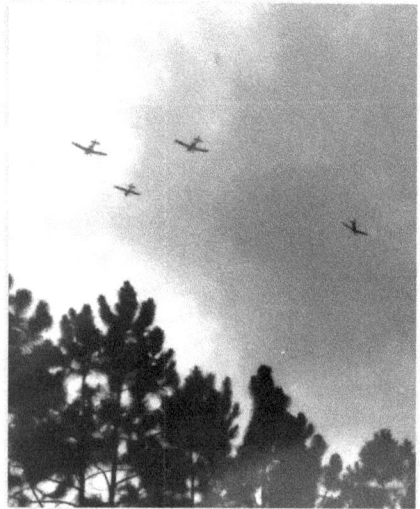

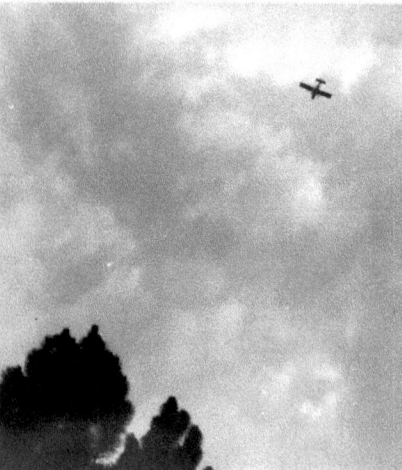

Chapter 28 — The "missing man"

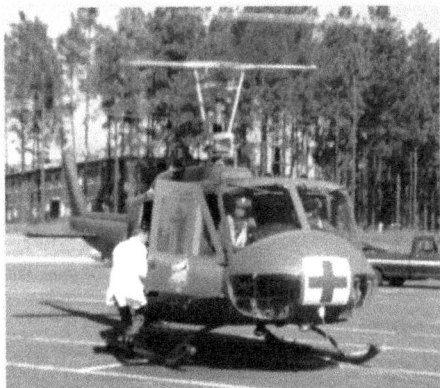

Chapter 29 —
Helping patient in helicopter
for emergency evacuation to
regional hospital

Chapter 29 —
Manning Christian
Academy Annual
Dedication

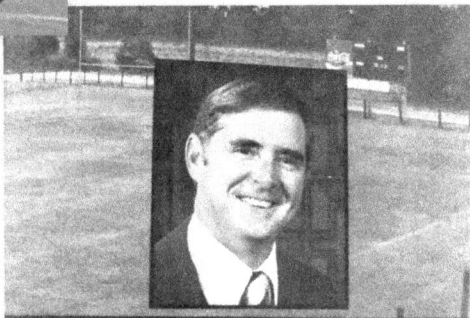

Dr. Robert Edward Jackson
1936-1978

Dr. Jackson served several terms on the Christian Academy Board of Trustees and also as President of the Athletic Booster Club. His energetic spirited participation in the school's athletic program as team physician and No. 1 fan was an inspiration to everyone. The instigation and development of a clinic for student trainers and coaches was an outgrowth of his concern for young athletes. The Scholarship fund was one of his pet projects resulting in a number of students being able to attend C.A. His love for God and Country was exemplified in his devotion to his church and the fulfillment of his military obligations. He never tired of extolling the virtues of patriotism and the privilege of being an American. This is the way we fondly remember him.

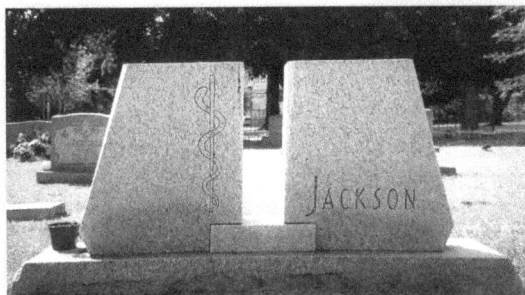

Epilogue —
Dad's headstone

Epilogue —
Dad's footstone

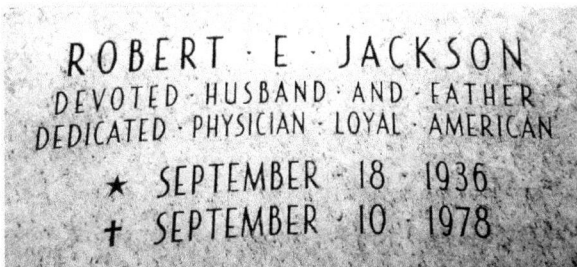

ROBERT · E · JACKSON
DEVOTED · HUSBAND · AND · FATHER
DEDICATED · PHYSICIAN · LOYAL · AMERICAN
★ SEPTEMBER · 18 · 1936
✝ SEPTEMBER · 10 · 1978

25

GIVE AND IT SHALL BE GIVEN UNTO YOU

Our family returned home from church one Sunday evening to find my dad already home with a young man from his Sunday School class, standing in front of his bedroom closet. Turns out this young man had accepted a call into the ministry and was soon departing for seminary in another state. Dad had about six or eight suits laid out on his bed, and the young preacher-to-be was trying on the suits one at a time. He and Dad were about the same size, so most of the suits fit him just fine. Pointing to all the suits on display, Dad told the young man, "Take them all. They all fit you so well."

Overwhelmed and speechless for a few moments, the young man stared at the suits with his mouth agape, finally responding, "Doc, I thought you were going to give me one suit, not eight. I don't know what to say." His eyes welled up with tears, and he just stood there with his hands by his side.

Then Dad looked at him with that serious look that he sometimes got, "I was once starting out in school with no money and no decent prospects. Nobody thought I had a chance of achieving my dreams, but God brought people into my life who believed in me and supported me. I'm the guy God has brought along to support you. I can easily buy more suits, but it will be years before you will be able to." Reaching into his wallet, he pulled out several $100 bills and stuffed them into his friend's front shirt pocket. "Now you go study and become the best pastor you can be. If you get into a bind, just call me. There is more where that came from."

Overcome with emotion, the young man reached out to hug Dad. They stood there hugging for a long time, with him crying and Dad smiling. Dad pointed at me and then the suits, and I knew immediately it was my responsibility to carry all of those suits out to that fellow's car.

M.R. Jackson and his children were subsistence farmers, growing and raising only enough to feed their large family, with a meager amount left over with which to purchase necessities. The brothers often referred to their father and themselves as "poor dirt farmers from Sammy Swamp." Nevertheless, they did so with a certain amount of pride in their heritage and in their father's and their own accomplishments. Being aware of their humble beginnings, M.R.'s offspring had a generous spirit and a willingness to help others who found themselves in the same financially disadvantaged state from which they all managed to escape by dint of education, hard work, and the grace of God.

Upon interviewing my first cousins for background information, a common theme emerged: the generous disposition of the Jackson clan toward others and one another. My first cousin Johanna related to me that she took a trip to Clemson to watch our uncle Scott play football. Her father, Dad's brother Billy, sent cash with her to help Robert and Abbot with college expenses, even though at the time he was barely getting by with his fledgling farm operation. Uncle Billy wanted to go to college and medical school himself, but at the time there were no funds for that. He became a sharecropper for Ms. Nina McFadden instead. He later became known as the one to go to for removing stitches and pulling loose teeth.

My first cousin Charlotte Anne told me that our uncle Scott provided employment for his brother — and her father M.R. (the oldest brother) — when he was older and in poor health, even though he couldn't really fulfill his work responsibilities or show up reliably for work. She was just starting her career in another state at the time and didn't have the resources to help her father. She said to me, "I will be forever grateful for Uncle Scott's generosity toward my dad."

Anne Nivens, another first cousin, said, "After my mother divorced and returned to Manning, our finances were really tight." She continued, "When I was in high school, Uncle Robert called me over to his office and gave me and my sister Beth a gift certificate to My Lady's Shoppe in downtown Manning. I was always too small for their women's clothes, so I gave the gift certificate to Mama and told her it was from Uncle Robert so she could have a new dress. Mama always smiled when anyone talked about Uncle Robert. She simply adored her brother Robert and was so proud of his accomplishments. I never told Uncle Robert that I did that [gave the card to her mom]."

"My mama always adored Uncle Robert, partly because she was so proud of him, and partly because he was always so kind to her," said my cousin, Beth Hinson Phillips. "When I was about twelve years old, I began to realize Uncle Robert had quite a few poor patients whom he visited all over the county on a regular basis. He told Mama about one particular family that was in desperate need of food and financial assistance, so one day we loaded up some groceries and drove down near the lake to take them some food. When we arrived, Uncle Robert was already there. The house was in poor repair. Sitting on the front porch was a young man who obviously had mental deficiencies. His face was terribly deformed, and he was playing with and chewing on tin cans. As we were delivering groceries, this young man's mother said to us, 'Dr. Jackson is the only person outside of our family who will put his hands on my boy. He's not afraid of my boy. He comes out to see me and my boy so we don't have to take him into town.' Then she gestured toward the roof of her house and said, 'He also put a roof on this house. God bless him.' My mama told me Uncle Robert put roofs on many houses around the county."

Once she got started, Beth had a number of stories to tell about her "Uncle Robert":

When I was the mayor of Summerton, I visited the home of an aristocratic woman named Jeanine King, who had traveled all over the world with her husband who was a military man. She said to me, "Beth, after retirement from the military we came back to my husband's hometown of Summerton. We purchased a home needing some renovating, and while working on the home one day, my husband passed out. Within an hour and a half, he died. The funeral home director, who was the coroner at the time, wanted to put the cause of death on the death certificate as 'unknown,' thereby preventing me from obtaining a military stipend. According to military protocol there had to be a definite diagnosis for cause of death in order to qualify for the stipend. I realized the coroner was not a trained medical person, and that he really couldn't help me. I was referred to Mr. McFaddin, head of the VA in Clarendon County. After explaining my situation, he immediately said, "You need to go see Dr. Jackson." Questioning him, I said, "Why would he help us? We are not his patients." To which Mr. McFaddin emphatically replied, "Just go see him." When I met Dr. Jackson in his medical office and explained my situation, he asked multiple questions about my husband's health and the circumstances surrounding his demise. He was willing to give a definite diagnosis on the death certificate, which allowed me to receive the military stipend. If it were not for that stipend, I would be working as a waitress in some restaurant. Perplexed, I inquired of Dr. Jackson, "Why are you doing this for me?" He simply responded with a smile and one hand on my shoulder, "Ms. Jeanine, if I were in your shoes, I would want somebody to do the same for my wife."

The year I won Miss Manning, your dad called My Lady's Shoppe and instructed them to provide me with the finest dress they had in my size. He said he would take care of all the expenses. I'm satisfied I won the pageant in part due to the beautiful evening gown he purchased for me. After winning, he was as proud of me as if I were his own daughter. During my reign, anytime I participated in any public event, he showed up to support me.

Kermit Holliday, Robert's X-ray tech, shared the following incident:

Doc really cared about the whole patient. One rainy day a patient [L.J.] came in and told the other patients seated on the couch that she was sick and needed to lie down — so they moved, and she did, in fact, lie down. When she came to the examination room, it was discovered that she was wearing multiple layers of clothing, all soaking wet. Doc asked her why she was wearing so much clothing and all of it wet? She told him that her roof leaked and everything she had was wet. After she left, Doc called a local contractor and had a new roof put on Mrs. J's home. Many times, he had patients who needed to go to MUSC in Charleston for treatment who could not afford the trip. He would see to it that they got to MUSC and would take care of their needs while they were there.

Once in high school, I was riding back to town from our lake house with my dad when he suddenly pulled off the lake road into the front yard of a wooden framed house with a tin roof, a small front porch, no paint, and a few chickens running around in the bare dirt yard. A black woman was sweeping the dirt yard in front of her house. On the porch sat an obviously mentally disabled young man, not in a chair but on the floor. When they saw my dad, they both broke into wide smiles. He greeted both of them with big hugs and kissed the mama on the forehead. She beamed like the early morning sunrise. He sat on the front porch with his long legs dangling off the porch and held hands with the young man who was her grandson. I learned that her husband had abandoned them, and she was raising this grandson and several other grandchildren all alone. She couldn't work because she obviously couldn't leave this grandson all alone. Dad inquired about their well-being, their finances, and their church. He teased her grandson and made him laugh out loud. It was obvious there was sincere affection among them. Before leaving, he leaned on his hip, pulled out his wallet, and handed her several twenty-dollar bills, at which point she began to weep and thanked him profusely. They all hugged again and then we were off.

As we drove away, I inquired, "Who are these folks?"

His response, "Oh, just two of my favorite patients. She is hard-pressed without a husband and no job. Her church helps her a little, and she receives a very small government check. I pay her electricity bill and groceries each month." He said that matter-of-factly with no hint of pride.

I asked, "She can't make it on her government check?"

He looked at me sharply and replied quickly, "Son, it's not the government's responsibility to take care of the poor. That's your responsibility and mine as Christian people. It's the church's responsibility."

I pondered that for a moment and asked, "Why?"

Without missing a beat, he said, "When the government supplies people's needs, they trust in the government and politicians. When Christian people take care of them in the name of Jesus, they trust in God. Big difference!" He had obviously thought about that a lot. I didn't really understand the full implication of that statement for many years, nor the full extent of my dad's benevolence, of which I've only mentioned a few examples out of many.

In 2019, I spoke at Greeleyville Baptist Church for their annual homecoming celebration. Afterwards a man came up to me, identified himself, and said to me, "Your father paid my way through college. I had no way to pay for my schooling. He believed in me, encouraged me, and paid my way." Tears began to run down his cheeks and he cried as he spoke. "I work as an accountant now, but I could never have accomplished that without his generosity. I will be forever grateful." Then with a great big sob, he threw his arms around my neck and said, "I can't tell you how grateful I am." I was quite taken aback and really didn't know how to respond. In thinking about it later, I realized I shouldn't have been surprised, because that generosity on Dad's part was entirely in keeping with his character. It would have made Isabel Weinberg smile.

I am convinced that kind of generosity grew out of my dad's deep-rooted spiritual life. He was born again into the kingdom of God at age ten. He joined First Baptist Church Manning on May 6, 1945, and was baptized. After his baptism while he was changing into dry clothes, his family loaded up into the family car and promptly drove home, unknowingly leaving their newly baptized younger brother at the church. He had to walk five miles to Sammy Swamp all alone, pondering the implications of his new Christian commitment.

The Bible says, "Give and it shall be given to you, good measure, pressed down and shaken together shall men pour into your lap." My dad was known for his generous and charitable disposition. One might attribute that to his less-than-ideal financial beginning. However, we all know folks who started out poor and like Ebenezer Scrooge have no charity in their hearts. Their attitude is "Get all you can, can all you get, sit on the lid, and poison the rest." Not so with my dad. I'm convinced that his generous, giving spirit emanated from his genuine Christian conviction that we can't out-give God — that the more we give, the more He gives to us. He had a heart of compassion and cared deeply for those less advantaged than himself, and he had confidence in God's supernatural ability to continue to pour into his lap if he just kept on giving.

Coming from humble beginnings, this dirt-poor farm boy from Sammy Swamp became a prosperous and influential physician in his hometown. Living in one of the poorest counties in one of the poorest states, he never forgot his origin or his Christian beliefs. He gladly became a conduit of God's grace and generosity in the lives of many impoverished patients. "Give and it shall be given unto you."

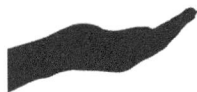

26

THE FLYING DOCTOR

Robert developed a keen interest in flying even before departing for Southeast Asia, where he participated in over ninety combat flying missions in multiple different types of small planes. He had obtained his private pilot's license only a short while before entering the Air Force. The Air America pilots often allowed him to fly the planes with their supervision, which only served to whet his appetite for flying. He wrote home to Abbot on September 6, 1966, "When we returned from Udorn with twenty-two units of fresh blood, the pilot allowed me to fly the plane, which is almost like a Cessna 172. The pilot fell sound asleep and left me to navigate over the mountains and through the clouds. I came in right over the hospital and then woke him up. It was a really good flight."

After returning to the States, he took additional flying lessons at England Air Force Base in Alexandria, Louisiana, in order to become instrument-rated. His passion for flying small planes was fully aflame. When he returned to private practice in South Carolina, it wasn't long before he purchased his first plane, a Grumann American Traveler, a yellow four-seater, low-winged aircraft with a retractable canopy. Having acquired my private pilot's license in high school at Dad's insistence, I enjoyed piloting that aircraft as well. I took my private pilot flying test on my seventeenth birthday in 1972, which meant that unless some other seventeen-year-old took his/her flying test on the same day, I would have been the youngest pilot in the country for a short period of time. I took my flying test in an ancient 175 Cessna, which was quite unwieldy but very forgiving.

I performed turns about a point, stalls, spins, and touch-and-go landings for the instructor. He never said a word, but I could tell he was incredulous that a seventeen-year-old-boy performed so well in such an awkward-flying machine. On my last landing, the wheels touched down so softly, they didn't even screech when touching the tarmac. At that point, he burst out laughing and started clapping. I didn't even smile. I just acted like I did that every time I landed that big old 175 Cessna. Dad loved my accomplishment, and we loved to talk about flying together. It delighted him to no end to come home from work and find me poring over a *Flying Magazine*.

Dad quickly upgraded to a Cardinal RG, a high-winged Cessna that flew at 190 knots. I also piloted that plane, but only with Dad in attendance. I once landed it at Clarendon Memorial Airport after dark; I must say, it was another very smooth landing.

Dad congratulated me and then asked, "When was your last night landing?"

I replied, "Dad, that was my first one!"

He nearly jumped out of his seat. "You mean you just performed your first night landing in my nearly new Cessna?"

"Yes, sir, I did," I replied smugly.

He regained his composure and responded, "Well, you performed admirably." I could tell he was really proud, and later I heard him bragging to the fixed-base operator after we off-loaded our gear.

Later, he upgraded to a used Beechcraft Bonanza, a real Cadillac of an airplane that flew at 220 knots. He flew at every opportunity. He often came home on his afternoon off, sat on the couch for five minutes, then full of restless energy, he would say, "Come on, boy. Let's go flying," which was music to my ears. Ten minutes later, we were at CMA, warming the engine of his airplane. We spent many lazy afternoons tooling around the county or performing touch-and-go landings.

He flew to Clemson football, basketball, and baseball games every chance his schedule allowed. Once he flew to Omaha, Nebraska, with my brothers and me to watch the Clemson baseball team play in the College World Series. (I later discovered that one of my Spartanburg patients was a behind-the-plate umpire at that particular series.) To this day, my brothers and I still talk about the fun we had on that trip. On another occasion, he flew us to the Florida Everglades, where a friend of his was a park ranger. His friend took us on an extended airboat ride through the Everglades National Park. Afterwards, the four of us went out to eat that night. We all bought yo-yos and threw them while we stood in line to watch the initial showing of *The Sting* starring Robert Redford at a theater in West Palm Beach.

When I attended Clemson University, Dad flew his plane to the small city airport where I picked up him, my mom, and their guests, and drove them to the football stadium for home games. As a lover of all things Clemson and a longstanding IPTAY donor, he had VIP parking right at the stadium gates. After the games, I returned them to the airport; then, he and I would compete to see who got home first — Manning for him, and the dorm room for me. All I had to do was negotiate the after-game traffic for approximately four miles, park my car, and walk a half mile to my dorm. He had to fly 200-plus miles, park his plane, and then drive ten miles to our home. When I arrived at my dorm room, my roommate would always say, "Your dad called. He's already home." He could fly in his plane at 6,000 feet while listening to the football games on the FM radio in forty-five minutes time, covering all 200-plus miles, faster than I could negotiate only four miles in the traffic. It always left me quite exasperated.

As much as he loved to fly and as much as he loved Clemson, his patients came first — as illustrated by a story shared with me in 2019 by one of his former patients after I spoke at a Greeleyville church:

I was pregnant with my first child and due to deliver any day. I got wind that your dad was planning a trip to Clemson for a football game in his airplane. I was already in the hospital due to high blood pressure but not in labor yet. He came by to check on me before leaving for the ball game when I had my first contractions. He assured me that his partner would take good care of me if I actually went into labor that day. I looked him straight in the eye and said, "Dr. Jackson, don't you leave me here all alone with my first delivery."

Your dad didn't hesitate. He just said, "I'll be right here with you." He called your mom and his friends and cancelled the trip on the spot. Later that afternoon, he delivered my baby girl.

Then she stood to one side and introduced me to her daughter with great big tears in her eyes, saying, "And this is that baby girl! Your dad was the best doctor ever. I miss him even today."

Through misty eyes, trying not to embarrass myself and choking down a sob, I muttered softly, "Yes, ma'am, don't we all."

The following is an excerpt from an article in *The Sumter Daily Item*, a Sumter, South Carolina, newspaper written by Mac McLeod, the paper's sports editor, on Thursday, December 11, 1975, entitled "Faith and Trust":

Every day we place our trust in the hands of someone or something, whether it be in sincerity of someone indicating a turn at an intersection or our car getting us safely to work. Trust in others is a part of life.

But perhaps never do we place so much faith in another individual as we do in an airplane pilot. Once you buckle up in a plane seat, you are at the total mercy of the ability of that one man to take you from the ground into the heavens and bring you back down in one, breathing piece.

It's a big responsibility, and although there are many who take to the airways, there are only a small majority who are totally capable. DR. ROBERT JACKSON IS A MEMBER OF THAT SMALL GROUP.

Dr. Jackson called me one morning last year from his Manning office and asked if I would like to fly with him to Tennessee to see Freddie Solomon play a game. I was more than happy to go see Fred play, but since I didn't know Dr. Jackson, I was a little hesitant.

If there is one person you should know, it is the man sitting at the controls.

As it turned out, the weather was bad, and Dexter Hudson ended up driving us to Chattanooga.

Then several weeks later, I got up my nerve and decided to call Robert and see if he would like to fly to Tampa, Florida, to see Solomon perform. He said he would, and I got the tickets. We set the time. He would pick me up at the Sumter airport on Saturday morning, and we would fly back the following Sunday.

Well, I checked every weather station within 100 miles all week long and even called Florida to check the conditions down there. I wanted to be sure there would be nothing but blue sky all the way down and back.

When Saturday rolled around, I was waiting at the airport, and shortly, here came Robert in his Cessna Cardinal.

"Mac, I'm Robert Jackson. Ready to go?"

We climbed aboard and Robert got ready to take off. He checked the gauges and went through a line of things. I was watching every move. I didn't know what I was looking for, but I wanted to be sure he looked at everything on the dashboard.

"OK, we're ready to go," he said, "but let me put my hat on."

That was all I needed.

"Every airline captain needs a hat," he joked, as he pulled out this white painter's cap with Manning Hardware Store printed in red across the back.

I laughed, he laughed, and we taxied down to the end of the runway.

"There are two things useless in life," Robert continued, "the
runway behind you and the sky above you."

A quick analysis of what he said brought home the message.

"This cat doesn't take any chances."

The trip was a wonderful one, and we made several more
thereafter, mostly to Clemson football and basketball games. He
would explain just about everything that was going on, and I grew
extremely confident in his ability to fly the plane.

But last weekend's trip to Miami iced the cake.

We had made plans several weeks back to see Solomon and the
Dolphins play O.J. Simpson and the Buffalo Bills. I got the tickets and
made the motel reservations, and Robert was going to fly the plane.

He had bought himself a new craft, a Beechcraft Bonanza, and
he was anxious to take it on a long trip.

Dexter was going on the trip, and Saturday morning we met
Robert at his office in Manning.

"Looks like good weather," he said, greeting us, "but we might
run into a little rain. We are going to Charleston and pick up a friend
then go straight to Miami."

"Let's go."

The flight to Charleston was uneventful, except for a small
rain shower, which doesn't bother Dr. Jackson at all. We put down,
picked up his friend, and after another weather check, took off.

THAT'S WHEN THE FUN BEGAN.

From 400 feet all the way to 8,000, it was a steady downpour
and all you could see out the windows was white. I couldn't see, and
I knew Robert couldn't see, but all the while I watched him keep his
eyes glued to the instruments — and, just for assurance, I would
take a glance at that painter's hat.

As long as he's got that hat on, everything will be fine. We
broke out of the storm around Jacksonville, and the rest of the

flight was beautiful.

As Sunday's game progressed, clouds started building in the east, and I kept my eyes more on them than on the game. I had almost enough money to spend another night in Florida if necessary.

By the time we took off, the sky was again beautiful, and south Florida was a magnificent sight from 9,000 feet at night.

But the closer we got to home, the worse the weather got, and finally, Charleston was so socked in, we had to land in Savannah and spend the night.

"DISCRETION IS THE BETTER PART OF VALOR," Robert explained as we climbed from the plane. One more mark for the good doctor.

Monday morning didn't look much better than Sunday night, but Robert checked with Charleston and said we could make it, so we took off.

Clouds engulfed us at 400 feet, but the painter's hat sparked my confidence, and at 3,000 feet we broke into a beautiful, blue sky. But that was only a minor part of the trip. I knew we had to land sometime, and, sooner or later, we would have to go back down through that white ocean of clouds. Sure enough, about thirty minutes later, Robert said we were going down and started the descent.

Outside you couldn't see a thing. NOTHING. And for a while even the painter's hat lost some of its appeal.

Down. Down. To the right. To the left. Up. Then back down. Back to the right. Then back to the left. We were getting close to the ground, and I wanted to see that runway. All the while, Robert continued to talk to the ground and watch those instruments. I couldn't talk to the ground, but my eyes never left the dashboard.

FINALLY, THERE IT WAS. THE CHARLESTON AIRPORT. If I hadn't thought it would have brought some staring eyes, I would have kissed Robert.

"Nothing to it," he chuckled. "Now let's get to Manning."

Once again it was back into the clouds. This time I knew there wouldn't be a radio on the ground to talk to, so Robert explained how he would catch a radio beacon out of Vance, take a ninety-degree turn, and break out of the clouds right over the Manning runway.

After the job he had done in Charleston, I didn't doubt him for a minute.

Finally, we started down, and the first thing he said was, "Let me know when you see the ground."

With one eye on the clouds and the other on the altimeter, we descended. Nine hundred, seven hundred, five hundred, four hundred, and still no solid soil. Then at three hundred feet there it was — that war-torn, hatred-filled, starving, depressed piece of beautiful trees, water, and hard ground called earth.

BUT THERE WAS NO MANNING RUNWAY. We had popped out over Potato Creek and were flying right under the clouds. Robert made a turn and started for where he was certain the strip was.

And sure enough, there it was. He put the plane down, and we simply all walked off as if there was nothing to it.

Actually, there hadn't been. During the entire flight, Robert maintained his cool and kept his painter's hat in place — and as long as he keeps that hat, I'll fly with him anywhere.

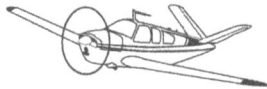

27

THE FINAL FLIGHT

On Friday nights, high school football reigns supreme in rural towns and urban cities across America — at least it did in the 1970s. This was, and probably still is, no exception in my small hometown of Manning. Located in a rural county of 26,000 people, the town still sports multiple football teams. Manning Christian Academy was one of them in the '70s. Dad absolutely loved football, as revealed in the words of his employee and my first cousin, Anna Lynn Floyd, "Uncle Robert told me, 'Anna, this is going to be my kind of fall. Clemson has a promising football season coming up. Richard is quarterbacking the Christian Academy football team, and John Reed is the running back.' More than that, he was excited about flying to Houston the following week. How quickly life can change."

Indeed, little did we know we were about to gather at the last football game we would ever attend with our dad. Our entire immediate family was at the game.

In September of 1978, Dad was a trustee of the academy and the physician for all of the athletic teams. His two younger sons, John Reed and Richard, also my brothers, were the running back/backup quarterback and quarterback respectively as mentioned previously. Every Friday morning at breakfast, he gave his sons the same advice: "Boys, run that ball with reckless abandon. If you get into a tough spot, just bow your neck and push through." Every Friday night, the good doctor tried to restrain himself from coaching and stick to doctoring, but the "struggle was real."

As usual, Dad showed up in his purple pants and gold shirt, the team colors of the MCA Deacons. With a bit of humor, one family friend said, "For another dollar or two, I believe Doc could have bought a pair of purple pants." On this particular Friday night, his face beamed with pride over his family. As his eldest son, I (Robin to family, and Robert to my college and medical school colleagues) sang the national anthem before the game began. My sister, Anne, and my mom, Abbot, sat in the stands. Both of his boys played well that night. He relished the fact that the entire family was together. (As a proud father, Daddy often spent time reporting on his children's accomplishments to anyone who would listen.) All in all, it was a great family night together, but none of us at the time realized just how precious this night would become to our collective memory. Oddly, we don't speak of that night much; it's both sacred and painful.

On Saturday morning, my path crossed with Dad's. He was returning from the hospital and met me leaving our neighborhood to return to Charleston for my second year of medical school. He signaled for me to pull over — then he pulled his own car over on the side of the road, jumped out, and bounded across the road with his usual energy and enthusiasm. Throughout my college years and my first year of med school, whenever I left home to return to school, Dad usually caught me in my bedroom while I packed my belongings. He invariably reached to hold my hand and commenced to praying over me.

This time, he knelt down in the road, stuck his hand through the driver's window, and grabbed my hand. Holding it with his strong, manly grip, he prayed for traveling mercies and for my success in my second year of med school. Afterward, we said our typical goodbyes; then he stood and turned around while I watched as he hurried back to his car — ever ready to move on to the next thing. Simultaneously, he turned toward home, and I headed in the opposite direction toward school — totally and blissfully unaware that these moments together and these goodbye words would be our last, and that this would be the last time I would ever see my father on this earth. His prayers over me spoke volumes to my young heart and now invoke some of my most precious memories of him. I can still see him bounding across the road and kneeling at my car door — all to pray for me.

The next day, as was his custom, Dad made Sunday morning rounds at the hospital. He met his sister, Eunice, at the hospital where she was working at the time. When he finished checking on his patients and signing off on his charts, she said, "Rob, please sing for me in church today."

He responded with excitement on his youthful face, "Sis, I'm flying to Houston today to a medical seminar."

"Well, who is going with you?"

"Abbot cannot go due to school starting next week. I invited Carl to go, but he has work responsibilities. So, it's just me," he responded with a smile.

"Rob, that's a far distance for you to go all alone," Eunice said with motherly concern in her eyes. "You may get tired and sleepy."

"Now, Eunice, don't you worry. I'll stop and rest halfway there. Y'all pay particular attention to my patient with pancreatitis. He should do fine."

As Robert turned to leave, Eunice spoke one last time to her baby brother: "Rob, that's a long trip for you to take to Houston today." A few of the nurses nodded in agreement.

With a reassuring smile and a pat on her shoulder, he said, "Sister, you fly low and slow, and I'll fly high and fast." Then he turned and walked quickly down the hall and out of her life forever.

The day was September 10, 1978. Dad left early on that hot summer morning to fly to Houston, Texas, to a Flying Physicians meeting, then from there to speak to a group of family medicine residents in Tennessee about the rural practice of family medicine. He had taken photos of our local hospital, the surrounding rural countryside, and the nearby recreational lake to help promote the rural practice of medicine in our community. Of course, he carried with him a doctor's bag full of anecdotes — both serious and humorous — to describe a country doctor's life. As he always did, he promised Mom, "I'll call you when I arrive at my destination. My ETA is 6:00 p.m. Texas time."

I can't say it often enough: Dad loved to fly, and he loved to fly his plane high above the earth where he could leave behind his daily responsibilities and focus on the challenge of flying his charted course. Slipping "the surly bonds of earth and flinging his eager craft through footless halls of air" persisted as one of his greatest joys in life. As he left behind the cares of his medical practice, he meticulously observed the rules of flying safety and, indeed, he often taught classes on flying safety to the pilots at McEntire Air National Guard Base. He completed his lectures by saying, "You can't use the runway behind you or the sky above you." This admonition encouraged pilots to leave plenty of room to maneuver and never take chances. He followed that maxim strictly.

"Are you sure you don't want to go with me? It's a beautiful day to fly!" Dad exclaimed to my mom with his normal zest for life and excitement for flying. That day he wore a bright yellow sport coat, one of his favorites, in keeping with his reputation as a sharp, classy dresser. In his early medical career, he was Mr. Conservative, always wearing dark suits, white shirts, and a thin black tie — until he attended a medical conference in San Francisco. To everyone's surprise, he returned with multiple brightly colored suits, multi-colored ties, and even blue and white shoes. He was the talk of the small town of Manning for weeks. It was a permanent transformation. The new suits perfectly matched his cheerful, sunny disposition.

"You know I can't go with you this time," Mom responded. "It's only the second week of the new school year. I can't afford to miss a week of school this early in the year. I promise I'll go with you to the South Carolina Family Physicians meeting in Hilton Head in November." Mom and Dad parted ways with a farewell hug and kiss, her going to Sunday School and him eagerly heading to Clarendon Memorial Airport to fly his newly uphol-stered Beechcraft Bonanza to Houston.

Arriving at the airport, he quickly but methodically ran through his preflight check, as every good pilot does — checking for condensation in the fuel tanks, observing for full and free movement of rudder and ailerons, running the engine up to full throttle, checking the brakes, magnetos and altimeter settings, and assuring that all avionics are fully functional. Hot and stuffy on that warm September morning, the cabin felt uncomfortable. Sweat ran down the back of his neck as he completed his preflight check and began to taxi out to the end of the runway. Lining up the nose of his beautiful, prized aircraft with the center of the runway, the white lines stretched out in front of him for nearly a half mile of runway. While he pressed both brakes, he pushed the throttles to maximum power. The plane strained to be set free like thoroughbred horses at the starting line. I'm confident he whispered, "Ride 'em, cowboy." Releasing the brakes, the Beechcraft Bonanza hurtled down the runway, pushing him back into his seat, a smile playing across his lips at the sensation of speed. The plane began to feel light in his hands. He pulled back ever so slightly on the yoke, and his craft was immediately airborne just a few feet off the ground. It gathered more speed, then soared free of the earth, banking slightly to the right en route to Houston, Texas.

In a matter of minutes, he achieved his cruising altitude and checked in with Charleston ATC (air traffic control) to verify his flight plan and to be picked up by their radar system. Free air-conditioning replaced the typical southern summer heat and humidity at that altitude. Looking down, he beheld a green and brown patchwork quilt of farms, pastures, roadways, rivers, homes, and churches. Above him was the vast blue dome of the heavens sprinkled with occasional white wispy clouds. To the right and left of him, there was nothing. He was all alone in that part of creation called "the expanse." Filled to the brim with the joy of commandeering his own flying machine, "he chased the shouting wind along on laughter-silvered wings."

Approximately three hours later, Dad landed at the Pine Belt Airport in Hattiesburg, Mississippi, where the flying conditions continued much as they were when he left Manning and where he refueled and purchased a grape juice. He contacted the McComb, Mississippi, flight service station for a weather update at 1307 CDT, and he received information of thunderstorm activity in southern Louisiana below his route to Houston. Dad acknowledged this and filed an IFR (instrument flight rule) flight plan to Houston via Lake Charles, Louisiana. He took off again at 1318 CDT (military time, also 1:18 p.m. CDT). The following excerpts are the actual transcript using military time instead of Greenwich Mean Time between Dad (N5642S) and the Houston Air Route Traffic Control Center (1R12 or 1R30).

After taking off from Pine Belt Airport, he climbed to 8,000 feet altitude and requested ATC (air traffic control) clearance:

1318:24	N5642S	Bonanza five six four two sierra, I'm just off Pine Belt IFR to Houston like to pick up an ATC clearance
1320:13	1R12	Bonanza five six four two sierra, you are cleared to the Houston Hobby Airport as filed climb and maintain eight thousand report reaching eight thousand
1320:21	N5642S	Four two sierra is level at eight and do you have any significant weather on your radar ahead of me right now
1324:14	N5642S	Four two sierra is level at eight and do you have any significant weather on your radar ahead of me right now

At this point, seeing thunderstorm activity ahead of him, Dad inquired of Houston Center radar if they were noticing any significant weather on his pre-filed flight plan.

1324:21	1R12	Four two sierra --- I'm painting weather around the Lafayette VOR, however, that's well past my area of coverage. I do show weather around Lafayette. It appears to be going north towards Alexandria. I don't know how far the line goes but I show no weather between your position and west of Baton Rouge about twenty miles
1324:43	N5642S	Four two sierra, roger. There is a pretty good buildup directly in front of me and like to deviate to the left just a little bit
1324:49	1R12	Four two sierra, roger. Deviate as requested approved

The Houston Center radar reported a fast-moving line of thunderstorms approaching the path of Dad's predetermined flight. He decided to deviate from his flight plan to avoid this inclement weather and was given permission to do so.

1426:18	N5642S	Houston, four two sierra
1426:20	1R30	Four two sierra, go ahead
1426:23	N5642S	The weather looks pretty clear between me and Coco now

1426:25   1R30   Ah just prior to Coco there is a line, however, ah, it's very narrow, very narrow line of weather but it looks rather heavy. Ah there's no other place you can go sir. You are completely surrounded unless you go back the other way.

My flying instructor always told me that small planes and thunderstorms don't "geehaw." My dad pretty much told me the same thing on multiple occasions. The standard operating procedure when confronted by thunderstorms: "Perform a 180-degree turn and hightail it out of there." Dad always said, "Discretion is the better part of valor," and "Eagerness to arrive at a destination will overcome a pilot's good judgment and end in a fatal accident!"

1426:40   N5642S   Four two sierra, roger

1427:58   N5642S   Four two --- four two sierra is in heavy weather going downhill

Dad had flown into the angry maw of an unforgiving monster. With a boiling black maelstrom reaching up to 20,000 feet, his little plane became caught in a violent roller-coaster — losing hundreds of feet in altitude in a single second, then regaining hundreds more the next. Like cannons, ear-splitting thunder concussed the little plane, threatening to crush its fragile metal hull. Lightning flashes erupted all around, reflecting off the blackened clouds in every direction and causing disorientation instantaneously. Lest vertigo overtake him, he dared not look outside at the heaving ocean of roiling clouds that grasped at the metal speck in its horrible, violent grasp. Focusing intently on his instrument panel, the ever confident, ever self-assured doctor realized that he was in serious trouble. An alien thing to him, fear began to wash over him like the tides of the sea.

1428:11	N5642S	Houston, you copy four two sierra
1428:26	1R30	Four two sierra, negative
1428:17	N5642S	I'm in heavy weather with heavy turbulence. I'm descending.

Unable to fly above the storm clouds that threatened his safety, he determined he must descend below the surging ocean of blackness engulfing him. The radar plat revealed two and a half minutes of erratic maneuvering, during which his plane executed a 180-degree right turn followed by a 270-degree left turn as he attempted to escape the boiling cauldron.

1428:20	1R30	Roger, ah what are you doing down there turn right sir ah you'll be out of it you've turned left directly into heavy thunderstorms
1429:05	1R30	Six four two sierra, what's your altitude
1429:07	N5642S	Four two sierra (unintelligible), seven thousand
1429:09	1R30	Roger, are you in a right turn now
1429:11	N5642S	Affirmative

1429:13	1R30	Roger, ah (unintelligible) Victor two twelve to the west of Alex would be your best route turning left put you right into the heavy stuff
1429:55	1R30	Five six four two sierra, you should be coming out of it in just a moment. What's your heading?
1430:00	N5642S	Four two sierra's in a spin. I'm going …
1430:21	1R30	Five six four two sierra, what is your heading sir
1430:34	1R30	Five six four two sierra, Houston
1430:38	N5642S	Four two sierra I'm on three zero zero [degrees]
1430:40	1R30	Roger, maintain heading three zero zero. You should be out of it in just a moment
1431:57	1R30	Five six four two sierra, what is your heading now
1432:02	1R30	Five six four two sierra, Houston
1432:09	1R30	November five six four two sierra, Houston

1432:19	1R30	November five six four two sierra,
		Houston

1433:35	1R30	Five six four two sierra, Houston

The official accident report of the National Transportation Safety Board indicates that at 2:30 p.m. CDT, Pilot Jackson reported he was in a spin. The controller requested the aircraft heading, and Pilot Jackson replied, "Three zero zero."

After that communication, Dr. Robert Jackson's Beechcraft Bonanza dropped off the radar.

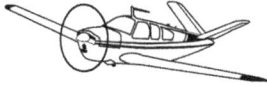

28

THE SEARCH

"Why hasn't he called me by now? He always calls me as soon as he checks into his motel." Peeved by the late hour without a call from Dad, Mom looked once again at the clock — 12:30 a.m. "Maybe he went to supper with his pilot friends. It's only 10:30 p.m. in Houston. I'll call his motel before I go to sleep."

"Has a Robert Jackson checked into your motel?"

"No, ma'am, there is no Jackson checked in at all."

Concern began to creep around the edges of her consciousness. She made more calls, beginning with the FBO (fixed base operator) at Clarendon Memorial Airport. Bill Stoia was asleep, but his wife suggested Mom call Charleston Flight Control, who then referred her to Houston Flight Control. Houston Flight Control reported a communication with Dad's plane and directed her to contact Scott Air Force Base in Illinois, where a search-and-rescue operation was located.

"This is Abbot Jackson from Manning, South Carolina. I am inquiring about my husband's airplane, Beechcraft Bonanza N5642S. Houston Control referred me to you."

"Yes, ma'am. Our last communication was at 2:30 p.m. CDT yesterday. We dispatched a search-and-rescue helicopter immediately, but the fog at ground level was too thick and they had to return to base. We will resume our search in the morning if we don't hear from the pilot by then. There are numerous landing strips in the area. Most do not have communications. He could easily have landed safely but be without means of communication."

The growing fear suddenly escalated into a paralyzing panic. Her mind was screaming, *Why didn't someone call me? Why do I have to find out at 12:30 a.m. in my bedroom all by myself from a man who must have ice water in his veins, judging by his businesslike manner?*

Mom crossed the hall and awakened John Reed (seventeen) and Richard (sixteen). With a trembling lip and a quavering voice, "Your daddy's plane is missing. Let's kneel right here beside the bed and pray for Daddy — Daddy's safety."

Thus, we began the worst five days in the life of the Jackson family. John Land — a lawyer, state Senator, and Mom's brother — arrived soon and began to quite capably organize the events of the next few days. The fear in Mom's mind was rampant and running away now. The almost certain knowledge of a crash, or at the very least a forced landing, bounced off the walls of her frightened mind. She kept pushing this certainty away, but when she related the fact to her brother John, the truth of the dire situation crashed down upon her, and she broke down in a fountain of hot tears. My sister, Anne, and I — along with Mom's mother — were notified, and the long, heart-rending vigil began.

It seemed to be a bad dream, as we all paced the floor while Uncle John began making telephone calls. He spoke with Scott Air Force Base again. It was only then that Mom found out she had not been talking with Alexandria, Louisiana, but with Scott Air Force Base — the National Air Search and Rescue Station. Awakened by the early telephone call, Bill Stoia, the fixed base operator at the Clarendon Airport, finally got through and pledged to conduct his own trace and investigation.

Uncle John spoke with Colonel Robert Johnson and General Grady Patterson of McEntire Air National Guard Base where Dad was a colonel and the state air surgeon. They pledged their support in the search should it become necessary. Everyone to whom he spoke that night assured us of Dad's skill as a pilot and of his calmness when faced with a crisis or emergency. "If anyone could come out of this safely," they assured us, "Robert can. He can fly that plane, and he knows what to do in a survival situation." We all had faith in Dad's abilities, but as the hours crawled by with no telephone call from him saying he was all right nor any new information from the Air Force base, fear became a constant companion clutching our hearts. We imagined what might have happened, picturing events up to the point of the crash, but none of us could picture a crash landing. We could envision a forced landing on some of the flat lowland around Alexandria, but we couldn't figure why Dad had not gotten to a phone by now — twelve hours later.

Mom reminded us of his saying, "Never leave the plane if you have a forced landing. Rescuers can spot a small plane from the air much easier than an ant-sized man walking through the field or the woods." We alternated between hopelessness and confidence that he would be found alive.

Uncle John had called Dad's six brothers and two sisters who lived in the area and notified them of the missing plane. They all immediately came to the house and joined in the vigil. Our pastor, Dr. Paul Sullivan from First Baptist Church, was called, as well as Dad's partner, Dr. Jim Roberts, and his office staff.

Uncle John spoke continuously on the phone in his quest for information. He ascertained that the weather in Alexandria was quite foggy with marginal flying conditions, but that two Air Force helicopters and five fixed-wing planes, flown by the Civil Air Patrol, would search when the weather permitted. Colonel Johnson contacted England Air Force Base and offered planes and men to assist in the search but was told the Civil Air Patrol was in charge and had the search under control. He was informed that too many planes in the area would be excessively dangerous. Due to weather conditions and much to our frustration, it seemed that the CAP was only searching sporadically.

The entire extended family felt frustrated by not being able to do anything concrete. Bits of information trickled in. Someone told us that in one of his last radio communications, Dad had said, "I'm in a spin." Then a couple of minutes later, he had said, "I've got control of the plane at 2,000 feet. I'm going to …" and then faded from the airways. We also learned that the area where he presumably went down was thick woodlands, five square miles in area. Uncle Jehu, the sheriff in our county, had contact with the sheriff in Alexandria, who reported that on Sunday afternoon a plane had been heard which sounded like it was in trouble near the spot where they were searching. Additional information came in that men on horseback and foot soldiers attempted to hack their way through the thick, marshy woods, thus searching in addition to the planes and helicopters.

Monday and Monday night crawled by. Our home overflowed with extended family and friends. The emotional tension and frustration squeezed all the breathable air out of the atmosphere. Sad and serious faces stared at the floor and then fearfully at one another.

On Tuesday morning, we decided that John and Robert's brother Carl would fly to Alexandria to personally supervise the search and give us positive assurance that everything possible was being done. The Federal Aviation Administration branch in Columbia sent a six-passenger plane to transport John, Carl, and a personal friend, Morgan Sauls III, to Alexandria. Officials briefed them upon their mid-afternoon arrival; however, they found the day's search winding down. They called to report satisfaction with the efforts thus far, and they would personally participate in the search on Wednesday.

Prayerfully yet fearfully, we continued our vigil in Manning. The assembled group in our home had now expanded to include neighbors, close friends, as well as the relatives who had been with us since Monday morning. Kind friends had brought food and served meals. The news of Dad's missing plane had been on the radio and in the newspapers. Phone calls came in from all over the state — indeed, from all of the United States, where Dad had colleagues and contacts. Dad's office had been open, but also had been deluged with calls from concerned friends, patients and colleagues asking for news and saying they were praying along with us.

Churches in Manning, Sumter, Summerton, and Alexandria, Louisiana, among others, held prayer vigils for his safe return. Local ministers offered up prayers when they came to our home. Our nerves were frayed, our spirits low, and our hearts heavy as we tried to keep hope alive. Each of us would often quietly slip away to the privacy of our bedrooms to fall on our knees to cry out to the Lord for the safe return of our sweet father and husband.

About 4:30 a.m. Wednesday, Mom awoke from a pill-induced sleep with a feeling of calmness. She had distinctly heard a voice saying, "They will find Robert today. Be at peace." Relief flooded her heart, and she came into my bedroom to share this with me. We prayed together, and then Mom returned to her bed for a few more hours of uneasy sleep. She told me that she had not dreamed for the past two nights as a result of the sleeping pills she had agreed to take so that she could make it through the days. She wasn't even aware who was answering the phone or taking care of the household chores.

When Mom arose on Wednesday morning, she was still quite calm and assured — although several times during the morning, she was struck with the thought that her dream had not assured her that Dad would be found alive, just that he would be found. Her calm was contagious, as everyone seemed to relax a bit. My brothers John Reed and Richard went to football practice, since they were necessary for the practice session.

Uncle John called a couple of times to report that the planes were methodically searching the five-square-mile tract of woodlands so dense that a downed plane could easily be overlooked. One thing that had puzzled us all along was why the plane's emergency locator signal had not been activated. Other pilots we knew had speculated that either he had made such a soft landing that it had not activated — or it was in the marshy ground, and he couldn't get to it in order to activate it. In the back of our minds was also the notion that he was injured and could not get to the emergency signal. We knew rain would have prevented his ability to signal with a fire. A report of an emergency signal being heard in a distant location, shining a momentary ray of hope, proved to a be a false alarm.

As the afternoon wore on, the tension returned as we began to wonder if Mom had only imagined hearing the message in the night. Dad's brothers and sisters had been in and out during the day, but most of them were present when the telephone rang at 5:00 p.m. Mom had not been answering the phone, but for some reason she picked up the receiver. It was John calling from Alexandria. He hesitated, then asked, "Abbot, are you ready?" She knew then what he was going to say. As we all watched frozen and expectant, Mom's shoulders slumped and tears slipped down her face as she silently listened to John's report. Aunt Marie was on another receiver. She announced for all to hear, "Robert's dead."

The plane had crashed about 300 yards from a meadow and about half a mile from a highway. Although the search planes had flown over the site many times, the woods were so dense that even now they had caught only a glimpse of the sun glinting off metal. When the planes turned to fly back over the spot, they lost sight of the downed plane again. The plane could only be seen at a certain angle with the sun shining on the metal of the wing. Helicopter pilots were called to hover over the crash site until ground crews could make their way to the crashed plane two hours later. Daddy was found dead, still strapped in the pilot's seat and gripping the controls. It appeared the plane was headed to a nearby clearing, but the plane's wheels had clipped the tops of tall pine trees and gone in nose down, plowing into the ground among the trees. The motor drove into the cockpit, causing severe head and internal injuries. Dad was eight days shy of his forty-second birthday.

The only two questions Mom managed to ask were, "Did he die instantly, and are you sure the plane didn't burn?" When she received those assurances, she handed the phone to my aunt Marie Land and stumbled off to find her children. We all hugged one another as fountains of tears flowed from our broken hearts. Through the fog of grief, I could hear the dam breaking behind me as Dad's older siblings let loose a week's worth of pent-up emotion and unbridled sorrow. When the emotional torrent subsided, my mom, though broken and grief-stricken, turned to Pastor Sullivan and with strength of character asked him to please say "a prayer for all of us."

Later Wednesday night, Aunt Marie, who had kept information straight for the last three days, informed us that John, Carl and Morgan would fly into the Clarendon County Airport in the wee hours. Our father's body would return by chartered plane around 8:30 a.m. Thursday morning. Bob Lee, our next-door neighbor, kindly transported our family to the airport to escort Dad's body to the funeral home. Finally seeing the flag-draped casket drove the truth home: We would not see Dad again on this side of heaven. Everything was so surreal, as our caravan escorted the hearse in front of the Clarendon Memorial Hospital where the flag was flown at half-staff in honor of its Chief of Staff, and past his office — a place he had loved with a passion akin to his love for his family. The bitter reality settled heavily upon our hearts, and none of us could find anything to say as we stared silently at the rear of the hearse containing the mortal remains of our beloved father. With a somber finality, we all realized that he would no longer come bounding in the back door with his quirky Jackson smile. We understood that the Sunday evenings after church of laughter over Mom's bacon and eggs were over. No longer would he "fling his eager craft through footless halls of air ... on laughter-silvered wings." It was many months before the laughter returned to our household.

The rest of that day was pure torture; however, making arrangements for the funeral was simplified by Dad having recorded his wishes, even listing pallbearers and hymns to be sung. Of course, as an active member of the South Carolina Air National Guard, he requested a military funeral because his love for the military ranked with his love for his medical practice. Interestingly, he had recently taught a Sunday School class on death and dying, in which he had challenged his class members to be prepared for the inevitability of death. As part of his class assignment, he had challenged them to write out their own funeral plans. Practicing what he preached, he had a file that included all of his wishes for his own funeral.

I assigned myself the responsibility those few difficult days of answering the front door of our home. A constant stream of friends, neighbors and church members visited to convey, initially, their hopes that all would turn out well — and, later, their condolences. Most everyone was long-faced and sorrowful. Manning the front door was an emotionally difficult task until our good friend Leroy Phillips stood in the doorway, smiling. He opened wide his arms and nearly shouted, "Praise God! Robert's gone to Jesus!" My heart leaped with joy, and we hugged each other. Mr. Phillips stood by me in the adult choir at our church and had patiently taught me how to sing tenor parts. He was the only one to greet me all week with the joy that I felt in my heart on my father's behalf. Yes, I was mourning over his premature death, but I knew that he had gone on to glory. "To be absent from the body is to be present with the Lord." I believed that with all my heart. I was not conflicted in any way regarding that truth. His exuberant confirmation of my conviction blessed me beyond words, and, after all these years, it's the only greeting that I distinctly remember during that entire week.

The hour of the memorial service — 4:00 on Friday afternoon, September 15, 1978 — arrived on a typically hot, Lowcountry afternoon. The skies were blue with scattered clouds, but no rain in sight. It seemed the entire town's normal hustle and bustle was on hold so as to honor its beloved physician. We steeled ourselves for the most sorrowful experience of our lives. However, we had earnestly prayed for spiritual strength, as did many hundreds of friends who had prayed on our behalf. In answer to many prayers, God gave us grace, and we were able to make the memorial a true experience of worship and a dignified tribute to our dad's life — a life spent in service to others.

Our family was completely overwhelmed by the huge crowd attending the service at First Baptist Church of Manning. Friends and family filled the sanctuary and gymnasium to overflowing, and many others stood on the outside. Unable to get in, several hundred people went directly to the cemetery or reverently listened to the service by radio. Dad's military colleagues from McEntire Air National Guard Base marched in together in their full military dress — dignified and somber — to serve as the honor guard and honorary pallbearers. Many medical colleagues from Manning and Sumter also served as honorary pallbearers. His office staff sat as a group; John Reed's and Richard's teammates and coaching staff attended as a group; Mom's fellow teachers sat together; and many of the hospital staff sat as a group. My sister and I were pleased to see her college and my medical school friends attending as well.

Our pastor, Dr. Sullivan, and Chaplain Jerry Hammett of the Air National Guard presided over the funeral service, which began with the singing of the "Battle Hymn of the Republic" sung by Aunt Katherine, Uncle Jehu's wife. In his comments, Chaplain Hammett stated, "Robert Jackson wanted to be remembered in a certain way, as do many other people. However, most people will not be remembered as they desire to be. Robert Jackson will be — because in his brief forty-two years, he lived so much more than many who have lived twice his age. He lived his life energetically, he lived it with a zeal and a zest — and for that reason, I will remember him as a man who loved life, who loved a challenge, who loved people, who loved his family, and who loved his God. I will remember him as a man of faith. I will remember him as a man of laughter, a man of boundless energy, and unlimited stories. I will remember Robert Jackson, and I am sure he will never fade from your memories."

Before Pastor Sullivan spoke, the congregation sang Dad's favorite hymn, "The Lily of the Valley," which begins with:

I have found a friend in Jesus,
He's ev'rything to me,
He's the fairest of ten thousand to my soul;
The Lily of the Valley — in Him alone I see

All I need to cleanse and make me fully whole.
In sorrow He's my comfort, in trouble He's my stay,
He tells me ev'ry care on Him to roll;
He's the Lily of the Valley, the Bright and Morning Star,
He's the fairest of ten thousand to my soul.

Pastor Sullivan reiterated Dad's generosity, his patriotism, his dedication to medicine, his commitment to the local church, and his love for his family. He then asked the question, "What made him such an outstanding man, and why did he make such a contribution to the lives of others?"

He suggested, "The basic reasons for his achievements, his honors, and his contributions could best be found in an incident which took place in my study several weeks ago. Dr. Jackson was preparing to teach a Sunday School class and came by to ask if I had a copy of a certain poem, which he not only wanted to use for his class but also as part of his personal testimony. The secret of his greatness is found in these words:

I had walked life's way with an easy tread,
Had followed where comforts and pleasures led,
Until one day in a quiet place,
I met the Master face to face.

With station and rank and wealth for my goal,
Much thought for my body but none for my soul,
I had entered to win in life's mad race,
When I met the Master face to face.

I met Him and knew Him and blushed to see
That His eyes full of sorrow were fixed on me;
And I faltered and fell at His feet that day,
While my castles melted and vanished away.

Melted and vanished and in their place,
Naught else did I see but the Master's face.
And I cried aloud, "Oh, make me meet
To follow the steps of Thy wounded feet."

My thought is now for the souls of men,
I have lost my life to find it again,
E'er since one day in a quiet place,
I met the Master face to face.

Dr. Sullivan continued with these words, "The one distinguishing characteristic that sets man apart from the crowd is his personal knowledge and fellowship with Jesus Christ, the living Son of God, the Lamb of God who takes away the sins of the world. His testimony was that he had been redeemed, not by corruptible seed but by incorruptible — by the Word of God, which lives and abides forever.

"Not many weeks ago, Robert shook my hand, and holding my hand in his, looked into my eyes and said, 'Paul, I want you to know that I love the Lord. I know that I'm saved. Pray that God can use me for His glory.' So as hearts are sorrowful and heavy today, we can rejoice with joy unspeakable and full of glory, knowing the truth of the Word of God that 'to be absent from the body' for the child of God redeemed through faith in Jesus Christ 'is to be present with the Lord,' which the Bible says is 'far better.' "

As the hearse left the church, hundreds of mourning townspeople lined the streets between the church and cemetery, and downtown merchants stood respectfully in front of their stores — a heartwarming sight to our entire extended family.

At the cemetery, the service was brief. The American flag was folded and presented to Mom by General Grady Patterson. The jets from McEntire flew over in missing man formation. The guns fired in salute. The bugler played "Taps." A group of local pilots and their small planes flew over in formation, with one peeling off to symbolize the loss of a comrade, eliciting sobs from both family and friends. Unplanned, a single dove rose from a nearby tree and disappeared over the treetops. Written words cannot describe the depth and range of feelings for me — and probably most of us.

We each laid a rose on top of the casket as we departed. In my heart, though deeply saddened, I knew that our father was not a resident in that casket. The Scripture verse played over and over in my mind, "O death, where is thy sting? O grave, where is thy victory? ... Thanks be to God which giveth us the victory through our Lord Jesus Christ." Jesus said, "I am the resurrection and the life: he that believeth in me, though he were dead, yet shall he live." My father was a sincere believer in Jesus Christ and a serious follower of Christ's commands. I have no doubt that he lives, and that we shall see him again on the other side.

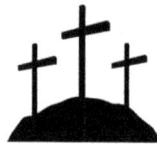

29

FOND MEMORIES

I was on call one weekend in my first year of medical practice in Spartanburg in 1985. While on call, I received numerous phone calls from sick patients, often necessitating a call to a pharmacy to phone in a prescription for some kind of medication. One Saturday morning, I called a pharmacy in Inman, South Carolina, and the pharmacist picked up, saying, "Revco Pharmacy."

"This is Dr. Jackson. I need to call in a prescription, please."

The phone line went silent. I waited, but there was no response. I repeated myself, "This is Dr. Jackson. I need to call in a prescription, please."

More silence. The hollow voice, now tremulous, inquired, "Who — did — you — say — you — are?"

Again — "This is Dr. Jackson."

The voice on the other end asked, "From Manning, South Carolina?"

Surprised, I responded, "Yes, sir. How would you know that?"

He inquired again, "Do you work at McEntire Air National Guard Base?"

"No, sir. That was my father."

The voice on the other end went silent once again, and I heard the distinct sound of quiet weeping — a kind of weeping I had heard many times as a family doctor while patients tried to regain their composure. In a broken voice, he said, "Son, I served with your father. He was one of the greatest men I ever knew. When I heard your voice, I thought I was hearing a voice from the grave. You sound just like your father. When you identified yourself as Dr. Jackson, it took my breath away. I couldn't talk."

Now it was my turn to be speechless. I didn't know what to say or what to ask. I called in the prescription, hung up and stared at the phone. I didn't ask his name, or how long he knew my dad, or in what capacity they served together. I was just totally blown away by the entire conversation, especially the depth of emotion provoked in a non-family member by the mere mention of Dad's name.

Similarly, my brother Richard remembers an incident from his job as a pharmaceutical rep:

My area director traveled with me as I visited doctors in my area of responsibility. Promoting a new blood pressure medication at the time, we were both excited about our new product, and doctors were intrigued by it. We called on a doctor's office in Sumter, South Carolina, where it somehow came out that I was the son of Dr. Robert Jackson from Manning. Suddenly, a black nurse threw both hands up in the air, and with unbridled emotion nearly shouted, "Lord God, I just loved Dr. Jackson. He was the sweetest man who ever lived. Lord, how I miss him, even unto today!"

Everyone, including myself, was stunned by her outburst. We all just stared at her until it became awkward, but she continued smiling this giant smile, radiant like a beacon, while rocking back and forth. Totally unaware of the awkwardness of the moment, she was caught up in the pleasant memories of Dr. Jackson, my dad.

I looked around at everyone staring at her, then stepped forward and gave her a big hug, and said, "We all miss him. He was the best."

Still smiling, she laughed, "He sho' nuff was. No doubt about it."

Back in the car, my boss looked at me with wide eyes and awe in his voice, and asked, "Who was your dad? That was a spiritual experience in there!"

Without hesitation, I responded, "Happens everywhere I go.

My dad was the greatest doctor who ever lived — barring none!"

Richard called on Dr. Roger Gaddy in Winnsboro, South Carolina, who told him the following over lunch:

I worked with your father one summer during my family medicine residency, when he called me in the middle of the night and asked me if I had ever participated in a breech delivery.

I immediately said, "No, sir, but I would love to!"

He responded, "Meet me at the hospital."

When we arrived at the hospital, there were complications with the delivery, requiring him to transfer the patient via helicopter from the rural Clarendon Memorial Hospital to the teaching hospital in Charleston. While we awaited the helicopter from Sumter, South Carolina, your dad quickly drove home, changed into his Air National Guard flight suit, and arrived back at the Piggly Wiggly parking lot with two flashlights in hand. When the helicopter arrived, your dad directed it to a proper landing using his flashlights. The laboring patient arrived by ambulance and was placed into the helicopter. Your dad jumped in behind the patient, leaving no room for me. The helicopter lifted off in a cloud of dust, disappeared into the night, and left me standing all alone in the Piggly Wiggly parking lot at 3:00 a.m., wondering what had just happened. To this day, I do not know how he got back from Charleston. Your dad called himself a "regular old country doctor." Trust me. He was nothing of the sort!

Further recollections by families and friends:

Uncle Ralph — As we worked and played together, I had no way of knowing that some years later my youngest brother, Robert, would become an outstanding physician. Occasionally, I stopped by his office just to chat a few minutes with him. As busy as he was, he never once failed to see me and always greeted me with a firm hand grasp and that boyish grin of his. He had a bounce in his walk and a seemingly endless supply of energy. Our conversations usually ended with a good joke and something about Clemson athletics. He always talked about his children, loved each one of them, and was very proud of them. He kept me informed of Robin's achievements at medical school and often invited me to see John Reed and Richard play football and basketball. One time I remember asking him how his daughter, Anne, was doing. He responded, "Ralph, that Sugar is something else." By that time, he had finished his cookies and Pepsi, so with patients waiting, I bid him goodbye with "I'll see you later, Doc." Those were the last words I ever spoke to him.

Uncle Jehu — In November 1977, I had a serious heart attack late in the night and Robert was called. I was brought to the Clarendon Memorial Hospital, and as I arrived, Robert was already there waiting for me. He examined me and had me sent on to Roper Hospital in Charleston. He rode in the ambulance with me, stretching out in the bed next to me, and every few minutes he would reach over and check my pulse.

I had a serious heart operation (four-vessel bypass grafting), and Robert made a number of trips to Charleston in his airplane to see me. I was always glad to see him and felt so much better knowing he was near. After leaving the hospital, I was seen at different times by Robert. I always felt that he was largely responsible for my recovery.

Aunt Katherine — On the day of Jehu's surgery, each of his brothers and sisters visited him in the hospital. They were allowed to go two-by-two into the coronary care unit for their visits. The nurses were amazed at the crowd. They were overheard saying, "They are running over in the waiting room." It was not long before the supervisor of nurses of the operating room came and offered her office to the Jackson family. We later learned that Dr. Hairston had requested this of her because there were so many of the Jackson clan. Suddenly, everyone missed Robert. Dr. Hairston called from the OR to tell Robert to scrub up and come into the OR to help sew Jehu up. No one could find Robert. We later discovered that he had gone to the medical college film library and was looking at films on some of the latest discoveries in medicine. He was always searching for new ideas. Fortunately, he arrived in time to get into the operating room and help with Jehu. It was a huge comfort to the Jackson family. Jehu recovered quite nicely, thanks to his brother Robert's fine care.

Dr. Peter Hairston — My feelings for Robert were, and are, genuine affection as well as respect and admiration. He practiced what I used to tell him was "frontline medicine," and he did it with an almost unique blend of expertise and compassion. He also did it in the face of considerable controversy — when his concepts, designs and needs proved too innovative for his "small town hospital."

Nevertheless, or perhaps because of all those things, he left a legacy of professional competence and demonstrated concern of which his family can certainly be proud.

I miss Robert. We used to talk almost weekly, and I always felt refreshed from our conversations. Almost reflexively, I still think of him on many occasions as if I could pick up the phone and find out about his latest adventures or a patient for whom we shared concern.

I'm not poetic, but I do feel my friend Robert passed like a comet through my life, and my days will be forever a little brighter for my good fortune.

Dr. Vince Mosely, Professor of Medicine Emeritus, Medical University of South Carolina — I had the pleasure of knowing Robert E. Jackson during his four years as a medical student and followed his career with much interest after his graduation in 1961. To me, he represented the best of two aspects of a physician — which are approaching patients' problems with a clear, scientifically trained mind, and the heart and empathy of a truly dedicated lover of his fellow man. Although highly intelligent and with an intellectual turn of mind, Robert was never arrogant, sophisticated, or pessimistic in his dealing with patients or his fellows. Though agreeable and respectful as appropriate to his company, he enjoyed joking and enjoyed bantering conversation. He often used his ability to relate humorous stories or events to illustrate points or facts, which he liked to make in times of serious conversation. In my mind's eye, I can still recall his bright face and lively eyes, and I can remember how he enjoyed the attention of others by his presence and speaking abilities. Robert, I am certain, will be remembered as a physician, community leader, gentleman, scholar, and one of those rare companions on life's way who is not only gifted in providing comfort for those in illness or distress, but also possessed of those qualities which made for a brighter and more enjoyable day for all who met with him.

Aunt Katherine — One of the big events of our life was the birth of our daughter Kay on October 6, 1971. When I found out that I was pregnant, Jehu and I discussed who I would use as an obstetrician. It was not a hard decision, because he and I both wanted Robert.

A few weeks after my first OB visit and learning the good news, we had another of those family suppers at Abbot's and Robert's lake home. Jehu and Robert began teasing me and saying, "We want you to tell everyone about your good news tonight." Abbot questioned, "What good news?" I then said, "You mean Robert has not told you?" Looking at Robert, she said, "No." Then I shared our good news. She replied emphatically, "Robert wouldn't tell me if my own mother was sick." Robert then said, "Everything in my office is confidential. No one learns any news from there." This was one of his admirable qualities. He never talked about one of his patients, and idle gossip was not one of his habits.

The day of arrival finally came for our beautiful baby. Robert allowed me to stay in my room during labor rather than go into the cold labor room. We almost didn't make it to the delivery room. The nurses called when we left my room, and it seems that it was only seconds before Robert arrived from his office across the street.

At the first sound of that little cry, Robert announced, "It's a girl," and in a few minutes he was telling me he was going to take the little girl out to see her daddy and grandmother who were anxiously awaiting the news in my room. He wrapped the little bundle from heaven up in a blanket and marched down the hall to my room. My mother often says she wishes she had a camera so that she could have recorded permanently the expressions on Robert's and Kay's faces when he came through the door. Mother recalls, "Kay was wide-eyed and gave the appearance of looking around the room. Jehu and Robert were bursting at the seams." For memories and moments like this, we say, "Thank you, God."

Dr. Sullivan — In Robert Jackson, I found a man of intense devotion to his ideals and principles in which he believed, and a man outstanding in every area of his life. He was a man who possessed great compassion and concern for his patients. He came from rather humble beginnings and never forgot the rock from which he was hewn. Remembering his beginning, he never forgot there were others in the same circumstances from which he had come, and he never failed to minister to those less fortunate. Despite his many accomplishments, he never thought too highly of himself. I saw him on one occasion literally give the coat off of his back to a patient who needed it. I think because of the privations he experienced as a young child that Robert enjoyed the simple things. I recall with admiration how he could have the greatest time in the world attending a church ice cream party and enjoy it as much as if he was sitting in the world's most expensive restaurant. He was a man so detached from the common concepts of greatness that he became great by being able to enjoy the simple things.

Out of his concern for the emotional and spiritual needs of families,

Dr. Jackson inaugurated a program at the Clarendon Memorial Hospital of Sunday morning worship services conducted by men of the First Baptist Church of Manning. Until his death, Dr. Jackson continued to supervise those services and to enlist the speakers and carried a major part of the burden himself. He was a member of the First Baptist Church of Manning. He had been president of the Brotherhood, he had been a Sunday School teacher, and he had taught in church training courses, a man constantly wanting to impart to others something of what he had learned — because in every aspect of his life, you saw, "Here is a man who cares."

I don't think in all my life I ever saw a more dedicated man, totally committed to medicine, and yet, in his dedication to medicine, he was one of those rare, strange individuals who was able to excel in many fields at the same time. He was an intensely patriotic American, serving in the Air National Guard, where he was Colonel Jackson. He loved his country, and he was an accomplished pilot who loved soaring the airways. He was outstanding in every area of his life, and yet, as outstanding a man as he was, the thing to me that most characterized Robert Jackson was compassion, love, care — however it may be expressed, it is concern for other people.

This stemmed from his personal faith in the Lord Jesus Christ. He said to me many times, "Pastor, I know that I am saved, and I want all of my life to count for God." In this man's care for others, I've seen him, because of the privation that he experienced as a young child, he so often, with guffaws, told me of a time as young boys when he and Scott and Carl, his brothers, had one pair of good socks between them and how they often watched for the laundry to go out to the clotheslines to dry so that whoever first saw the socks on the line could hide them so that he would have the good socks for Sunday School. Because of this, I think he cared deeply for those who had less of the world's goods than he had. I know of cases where he provided food and clothing. I've known him to put a washer and dryer in the home of a patient who was severely afflicted with heart problems and unable to provide for his family. He was a man who cared deeply.

The following article written by Ervin Duggan, a childhood friend of Abbot's, appeared in *The Washingtonian* in July 1980. Ervin served under President Johnson, headed PBS, served on the Federal Communications Commission, and most recently directed The Society of the Four Arts in Palm Beach, Florida:

"Who's the True Patriot?"

The two roads of our lives diverged after high school. He, the farmer's son, one of thirteen children, went to Clemson, the state land-grant college. I went out of state, to Davidson in North Carolina, one of those small private colleges steeped in southern tradition where the buildings wear ivy and the people wear blue oxford-cloth shirts.

After college, he went to medical school, and I came to Washington. He served for a while in the Air Force, then returned to our little town of Manning, South Carolina, to deliver babies, suture wounds caused by chain saws and fishhooks, and sit up all night with dying sharecroppers in their unpainted shanties. I did a stint in the Army, worked for a newspaper, a President, a Senator, a couple of Cabinet officers, and wrote a novel.

The real link between us was his wife, who had been my next-door neighbor and childhood playmate in Manning. Now and then, Robert would come to Washington for a medical meeting or an Air Force gathering, and he would stay with us. He would keep us up nights, regaling us with southern Gothic country-doctor stories — the 400-pound woman, for example, who had to be transported to the hospital in the back of a pickup truck and gave birth to triplets on the way.

He would tease me about losing my southern accent, and I would deny it hotly. But he was right in a sense: Without trying,

I had become urban, jaded, Washington, acquainted with finger bowls. His accent was so thick you could cut it. And he still walked as though he were stepping over furrows.

He was a southern-fried Republican who wore a flag pin in his lapel and — the last time I saw him — a bracelet bearing the name of a Vietnam POW. I was a liberal Democrat.

Suddenly, almost two years ago, he died. Flying his light plane to Houston to deliver a paper on the life of a country doctor, he encountered thunderstorms. He radioed that he was in trouble, then disappeared from the airwaves and the air. Days later, they found him in a Louisiana swamp.

I went home to his funeral. He had asked, in the careful instructions he left, to be buried in his Air Force uniform. The eulogy was offered by an Air Force chaplain. The crowds overflowed the Baptist church and filled the school gymnasium next door. There were flags everywhere. And the word used most often, other than his name, was patriotism.

I've been thinking about it ever since.

Patriotism. My patriotism is a complicated, Washington thing, full of subtleties and shadings, punctuated by question marks, not exclamation points. Knee-jerk patriotism, like fundamentalist religion, embarrasses me; embarrasses many of us in Washington. Glib about sex, we are curiously reticent about patriotism.

But we are patriots. We exhaust ourselves serving our country. We work long hours, write the budgets and the speeches, pass the laws, arrive late from the office at dinner parties where the most fascinating conversations take place: Why the Administration's MX missile program is a massive political blunder. What the Speaker said about Hamilton Jordan. Why the President really fired Mike Blumenthal.

Like theater critics, we survey the nation's latest performance

— a rescue mission to Iran, Muskie's trip to the summit — and sit in judgment, often harsh judgment. But we are patriots. Doesn't the theater critic still love the theater? What would you have us be — blind patriots, mindless patriots?

Mine, I tell myself, is a higher sort of patriotism: a quiet, intelligent, furrowed-brow patriotism. My patriotism asks hard questions, holds the country to a rigorous standard of conduct, does not give unquestioning assent. In my mind, I am constantly tapping Uncle Sam on the shoulder and saying, "Excuse me. Are you sure you're doing the right thing? I'm not certain I can go along."

My friend Robert Jackson asked few such questions, or none. His was the kind of patriotism that simply snapped to attention and saluted.

I knew, when he was in the Air Force, that he had volunteered for medical duty in Vietnam. I pictured him safely behind the lines, on a hospital ship offshore perhaps, or giving penicillin shots and VD-control lectures to troopers in Saigon.

After he died, I learned how it had really been. His wife sent me his papers, a jumbled heap of letters, records, clippings, and reminiscences by friends.

Sifting through his letters, I learned that he hadn't been in Vietnam at all. He had been in Laos.

He was punctilious about security; Laos was a secret — not officially a part of our war. When it was necessary to refer to a place or a person in his letters home, he would simply leave a blank space to be carefully filled in when he returned home. The place had been Sam Thong, an airstrip in a Laotian valley with a primitive hospital alongside, and a constant influx of patients: refugees, Americans with malaria, sick Laotian civilians, Laotian soldiers wounded in their war with the Pathet Lao, downed and wounded American flyers. He wrote home almost every day:

"When wounded are brought by aircraft to the hospital, the airplanes taxi up to the front door. The medics just push a stretcher up to the plane and offload the patient …"

"I drained four gallons of fluid out of an old lady's abdominal cavity this morning. I have before-and-after pictures of her … We were asked to discharge as many patients as possible today because a large number of casualties are expected to be in tomorrow …"

"Late this afternoon, the two worst facial injuries I've ever seen came in. One woman was struck by fragments from a land mine. Both cheek areas, eyelids, and lower lip were laid open, plus the left maxilla was broken and her right arm was fractured in three places. The other patient was a soldier who had been shot through the lower jaw …"

And all the while, the war was going on in the jungle right outside:

"It was a little after dark when I left the operating room to walk to Air America [the CIA-funded air-transport operation] for supper. Suddenly, I heard a shot ring out, but nothing happened … At night, it is a precarious walk around."

Meanwhile, I was in Washington, working on health and education programs in Lyndon Johnson's White House. I had come there as a green young staff assistant in 1965, in the euphoric aftermath of Johnson's landslide the previous November. That spring and summer, there had been a torrent of domestic legislation: It seemed as though there were bill-signing ceremonies every day — in the Oval Office, in the Rose Garden, in the East Room — with the President doling out pens by the handful to eager, cheering supporters.

By mid-1966, the atmosphere in the White House had changed. A pervasive, Vietnam-colored grimness settled over the place like smoke. And I noticed a curious thing: Even the people who were running the war — whose responsibility it was to plan it, prosecute it, and defend it — seemed to hate it. It was an unhappy time, for those who admired the President — and I was one of them — who cared about his programs, who felt his more ungenerous critics were dead wrong about the man.

One day the telephone rang in my office, and it was Robert, laughing. "I'm in the hospital at Andrews Air Base, but I'm OK. Come on out and see me."

I left the office and went to the hospital, where I found him sitting with his long legs dangling over the bedside, clad in blue military pajamas that flapped around his ankles. He had contracted malaria in the jungle. His skinny frame was skinnier than ever.

We spent the afternoon laughing and talking. He told me a string of wild stories from the hospital that I thought was somewhere in Vietnam: country-doctor stories, chain-saw and fishhook stories, land-mine and bullet-wound stories.

Amid the anecdotes, Robert said enough to make it clear that he didn't hate this war. He saw it as right and necessary. He believed the Pathet Lao and the North Vietnamese were murderers who served a murderous system — people who set land mines to blow up the faces of children and old women. He was glad to be home, but he was glad also to have done his part against his country's enemies. He had none of the ambivalence that I had seen in Washington and that I felt myself.

We shook hands warmly. I went back to the White House. The next day, they flew him home to South Carolina.

There, recovered, he plunged back into his doctoring. He built a gleaming family-practice clinic under some moss-hung trees in the town. He recruited nurses and paramedics and other physicians. He trained the local rescue squad, gave lessons on cardiopulmonary resuscitation, taught a Sunday School series on death and dying. When a freak spring blizzard suddenly paralyzed the South Carolina Lowcountry, he organized a rescue mission by military helicopters and went swooping about the county, airlifting stranded motorists and delivering babies in snowed-in homes.

In his spare time, he made speeches to civic clubs and medical societies, showing his slides from Laos — which he simply called "Southeast Asia." He would end with a little homily in defense of America and the war — the purest Fourth of July corn, all of which he believed.

Stories of his Asian exploits — of midnight rescue missions, all-night surgical marathons, miraculous recoveries — followed him home, along with a hail of medals and citations. The Air Force Commendation Medal. The Airman's Medal for Heroism. The Air Medal. The Legion of Merit. The Bronze Star. He was named Tactical Air Command Flight Surgeon of the Year.

And every week or two, he put on his uniform and drove to McEntire Air National Guard Base to fly and train with the pilots there. He could no more have given up his uniform than his white coat or his stethoscope.

He was an admirable man, but no plaster saint. He had a larger-than-normal ego. He was vain enough to love the publicity that his exploits gained him. He was a man whose lusty appetites sometimes got the better of him. He had a doctor's bottomless tolerance for human frailty, and he had his own frailties.

Once, just once, he let his flag-pin patriotism erupt into something other than tolerance. When an Army dermatologist at nearby Fort Jackson was tried for refusing to go to Vietnam, Robert exploded. He wrote a curt letter to the editor of the local paper, denouncing the man as a disgrace to his uniform and to medicine. He had trouble understanding such people, and he didn't like them.

I didn't like them either — from a distance. I found the war protesters strident and self-righteous, too quick to denounce their own country, too prone to ascribe the President's honest mistakes to evil motives. The trouble was that I kept bumping into my friends among the protesters — people who weren't strident or self-righteous at all, just deeply upset.

One day, walking to my office at the White House, I passed a little group of clergymen and seminarians keeping a peace vigil in Lafayette Park. One of them shouted my name and I stopped, caught short: It was a classmate of mine, a close friend. We talked awhile, and as I left, he called out: "If you weren't in there, you'd be out here, wouldn't you?"

I didn't reply. He was probably right, of course. But I was in there, and being there had changed the angle of my vision. Nothing would ever seem simple again.

Through it all, Robert Jackson and I kept in touch. I always saw him on my trips back to our little town. Always, we would argue about politics: He loved the flag, but he thought the federal government was evil incarnate.

Once, on one of his visits to Washington, we sat up late and argued about the war, the demonstrators, the resisters who had fled to Canada.

"What about them?" I asked. "Isn't theirs a kind of patriotism? They care about their country, but they believe, deeply and honestly, that the war is wrong. They're taking risks, too, aren't they?"

"Well," he finally said, "I guess they're entitled to their opinion."

At one point he raised his hand, then let it drop. "Your country is like your family," he said. "If somebody in your family gets in trouble, you help them. If your brother got in some kind of scrape, you'd help him, wouldn't you? You wouldn't just walk away."

It wasn't that simple for me, with my complicated, classically Washington, question-asking patriotism.

Years later, discussing the same questions with another friend, also a doctor, I made an analogy.

"Maybe people are patriotic the way they're religious. Some people practice their religion in a casual, half-involved way. Others are more thoroughgoing and radical. We call them saints."

"I'd put it a different way," my friend said. "There are born-again types, Jesus freaks who buttonhole people on the street, shouting, 'Praise the Lord.' And there are the Jesuits — people like Father Drinan who are very intellectual, cerebral, but who still give themselves to their religion — who still obey it." A good way of putting it, I thought. But where are the Jesuits of patriotism? Where are the people who are full of questions but full of devotion, too? Was Robert E. Lee such a man? Or George Catlett Marshall? My friend Robert Jackson was much less complicated, and I find myself envying him.

He died at forty-one, leaving a grieving town, a box full of medals, scrapbooks packed with press clippings and citations. And he left four children so deeply stamped with his values that they might have been tattooed. I went to his funeral in my Washington clothes and listened in wonderment as the chaplain described those values. Summed up, they sounded like Mother, God, and flag.

After the church service, we gathered at the gravesite. His wife stood at attention, and they handed her a flag wrapped into a tight triangle.

It was the purest, most ironic happenstance that Robert Jackson died as a civilian, piloting his own plane, rather than the way he would have preferred to die: for his country, wearing a uniform, flying a jet with a flag painted on the fuselage, or stitching up some wounded comrade in a field-hospital tent.

I don't know why he died. I don't know how he and I came to be so different — or why, despite our widening differences, we kept on liking one another so much. I don't know the answers to any of the questions that a life like his, and a death like his, set boiling in my mind.

I do know that his patriotism was the kind that, had I never known him, I would have labeled "blind" or "mindless."

But I did know him. And I believe his patriotism — simple and unquestioning as it was — was morally superior to mine.

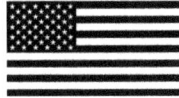

30

A Crooked Stick

My first cousin Johanna had just finished sharing with me a troubling incident that occurred in her family, then said, "Your dad came out to my house, sat down with me for several hours and just listened to me pour out my heart. Then he shared with me some very good advice. His presence was such a comfort to me. Although he was the youngest of the Jackson siblings, all of his brothers and sisters and their children looked up to Uncle Robert for wise counsel and medical care. He was like our family doctor and our pastor rolled up into one."

Indeed, Dad was often called on to provide medical care for the extended family. My uncle Billy took his wife Laura to the Medical College of South Carolina in Charleston (now the Medical University of South Carolina) to evaluate her chronic abdominal condition and weight loss. The specialists there gave a diagnosis and a treatment plan, including surgery. Billy thanked them politely, loaded Laura in his car, drove back to Manning, and consulted with his younger doctor brother. He wasn't allowing any surgeon anywhere to operate on his wife until Robert gave his second opinion and his approval.

Robert's sister Eunice recorded in her journal on May 10, 1979:

> Eight months today that Rob passed away. This has been a long time without him. I can't really feel that the hurt is any less. I still think of him so many times every day and during the night.

How could one man have touched so many lives? He possessed so many talents that other people never had. His energy was unlimited, his love, patience, understanding and great knowledge — his ability to diagnose and treat an ailing person — the leadership, wisdom that he possessed. Every day that I work at the hospital, some patient or employee tells me how much they miss Dr. Jackson. The love people felt for him is unending.

How great it was to have Rob for a member of our family. The consolation of having him to advise us about our problems, not only physical needs but anything that concerned us — he usually had a solution — an answer, an explanation. He advised us, he prayed with us, he cared for us.

Not only was Dad the extended family doctor and counselor, he was the organizer of family gatherings — which often took place at our home or our lake house. I recall many cookouts or ice cream churnings, followed by hours of storytelling by all of the brothers, who seemed to never tire of being together and enjoying each other's company.

As Johanna finished telling me her experience with my dad, she paused a moment then added, "Robin, your dad was the best doctor ever, but he was not a perfect man. Just remember that." I pondered that statement for a long time. Anybody who lives with someone long enough knows that individual is not perfect. None of us is perfect. The prophet Jeremiah tells us, "The heart is deceitful and desperately wicked above all things. Who can know it?" I was aware of many of my dad's warts and weaknesses. He had feet of clay just like the rest of us. However, thankfully, our foibles and failures do not define us.

I heard a preacher say one time, "God can strike a mighty good lick with a crooked stick!" If we think about it a little bit with a clear head, we realize that any time God uses any of us, He is using a crooked stick. Some of us are just a little more crooked than others. When your mama took a switch to your backside when you were a child, it didn't matter if it was straight or crooked, it hurt just the same! Likewise, God is able to use you and me regardless of our crookedness to accomplish His eternal purposes. Don't get me wrong. I'm not condoning iniquity, which literally means bent, crooked, or gnarled. I'm just saying that none of us is a straight arrow!

Now here's the catch. The Bible tells us that "there is no condemnation for those who are in Christ Jesus," which is a huge comfort for every one of us who have been born again into the kingdom of God. More than that, the Scriptures tell us that "God made Him who knew no sin to be sin on our behalf that we might be made the righteousness of God in Him." In layman's language, this means that God credits to our spiritual account the very righteousness of Jesus Christ. Even though we may still struggle with our three common enemies — the world, the flesh, and Satan — God has declared Christian folks to no longer be condemned and to possess the righteousness of Jesus Christ. By the grace of God and the power of Holy Spirit, we can walk in righteousness. Does this mean we will be sinless? No, it just means we can sin *less* as we go along our Christian pilgrimage. I'm satisfied that if God can use Moses the murderer, David the conspirator, and Paul the persecutor, then He can use those of us who have been washed in the blood of the Lamb, sealed by Holy Spirit, and had our names written down in the Lamb's Book of Life. We just have to focus on putting off the old man and putting on the new man, which is the lifelong process of sanctification.

I was close enough to my dad to realize he was troubled by his own sinfulness and struggling to sin less. He understood that, as a believer, Holy Spirit lived in him and provided spiritual strength to minister in Christ's name, which I believe he sincerely desired to do. My dad ministered out of a deep well of love for God that overflowed into the lives of others. That overflow was manifested as a genuine servant's heart to rich and poor, yellow, brown, black and white, old and young, educated and uneducated. He was "no respecter of persons" (in other words, he showed no favoritism).

The overflow of that deep well revealed itself in kindness, generosity, love of family, love of patients, love of church, love of country. He possessed a heartfelt compassion for his patients. He exhibited an overflowing joy in living life, in practicing medicine, and in loving his family. Out of that well flowed enthusiasm for everything to which he put his hands. No, Robert Jackson was not perfect. He was a crooked stick just like you and me. I heard him pray multiple times, asking God to use him in His kingdom's work. I am satisfied God heard his prayer and struck a mighty good lick with that crooked stick!

EPILOGUE

My father, Dr. Robert Edward Jackson, is forever young, forever youthful, forever energetic, always smiling that quirky Jackson smile, always ready to share a story so wild and crazy that you wonder, "Is he telling the truth or pulling my leg?" Most of us have the privilege of watching our parents grow old and observing how time and age steal away their youthful vigor and strength. We observe ever so slowly — and somewhat sadly — as they gather wrinkles, falter in their steps, and fade in their memory. Then we look in the mirror and realize the same, inexorable aging process has begun to affect us as well.

For some reason unknown to me, God chose to snatch Dad away as quickly as Enoch before time and age ever affected him. Scripture says, "Enoch walked with God; and he was not, for God took him." I doubt God negotiated with Enoch or gave him advance warning. He just exercised His divine prerogative and translated Enoch from this life into the next without death's dew ever settling upon his brow. I'm not suggesting that Dad was snatched away because of his righteousness, as was Enoch, or that he was translated without experiencing death. Nevertheless, I have questioned God's rationale from my human perspective. For you see, Dad was vital to our family — as is every father. He was integral to the medical community in our small town. More than anything and what disturbs me most, he was on a spiritual growth curve. The last summer before "God took him," I worked in his medical office — a blessing and a gift from God to me, to both of us. I spent long hours with my dad, riding with him and just talking about life. We talked about the Lord and about our common spiritual journeys, and we discussed the hard questions of medical ethics. I could tell Dad was curious about many spiritual topics and seeking answers, many for which I was too young to provide a satisfactory answer. Pastors would call that "seeking the Lord," and God promises that "those who seek Me will find Me." So why didn't God honor him as an essential player in our family and our community? Why didn't He allow him time to "seek and find"? Why couldn't we grow old together, practice medicine together, raise my children together, and go on medical mission trips together? Why is he not here to listen to me tell the wild and crazy things that happen in my medical practice or about the adorable things his grandkids said and did today?

My dad would be extremely proud of his children, his grandchildren, and his great-grandchildren, of which there is a "whole passel" of them. He was always proud of my mom. We could tell that when he held her hand at the dinner table and stared lovingly into her eyes. He would still be proud of her. She is a strong and courageous woman who takes care of all her family and her longtime friends. I don't know why Mom and Dad aren't sitting in rockers side-by-side, holding hands and watching reruns of Clemson championship football games. I don't know why my brothers and I aren't playing golf with Dad on Sunday afternoons.

There are lots of things in this life that I don't know, but this one thing I do know. If Robert Jackson could speak to us now, he would say, "Life is brief and uncertain — like a vapor. Get your spiritual house in order and trust in the Lord." When I get to heaven, after I've spent 10,000 years worshiping Jesus, I plan to ask Him, "Why, Lord, why?"

◆ ◆ ◆ ◆ ◆

After Dad finished suturing a laceration on one of his patient's forearms, he stripped off his gloves and left them on the surgical tray with his other instruments and surgical supplies. As he quickly left the room, he instructed his patient, "Keep the wound clean and dry. Change the bandage every day. Come back in twelve days, and we'll take out the stitches." With a pat on the shoulder and a smile, he was out the door and on to the next patient. Before the nurse came in the exam room, his patient reached up to the surgical tray and grabbed a gauze pad and slipped it into her pocketbook.

Twelve days later, she returned for the suture removal. The wound had healed nicely without any infection. Both she and her doctor were pleased. Before leaving, she inquired, "Dr. Jackson, do you have any more of your healing cloths?"

Looking at her perplexed, he smiled and said, "Excuse me?"

"Do you have any more of your healing cloths? I got me one off that tray after you sewed me up. I rubbed it on all of my sore joints, and, Lawd, do it make them all feel better!"

Realizing immediately what had happened, he grabbed several four-inch gauze pads and presented them to her, saying, "I prayed over these especially for you." She left beaming with delight.

At supper that night, Dad looked at my mom seriously and said, "I've decided that I am going to start selling healing cloths."

Mom looked at him with consternation for a moment, then laughed, "Pshaw, Robert, you're full of yourself."

Serious as a mortician selling caskets, he never smiled. He just kept on with, "I could get white handkerchiefs, and monogram Dr. Jackson's Healing Cloths on them and sell them in the Piggly Wiggly parking lot on Saturday mornings." His eyes started to crinkle, and his lips started to turn up. "I could get some teenage girls to clog and a little band to play music." He was all smiles now and getting really wound up, his voice getting louder and more excited. "I could put a pair of praying hands on one top corner, and the American flag on the other. We'll put a Christian flag on another corner!" By now he was slapping his thigh, leaning way back in his chair; then he leaned over and grabbed my arm and nearly shouted, "Then we'll put a Clemson tiger paw in the last bottom corner. Hey, Bo, what do you think about that? Do you think that will sell?"

All of us kids were excited. We could see it happening. Dad had tears streaming down his face, and he was laughing so hard he had to hold his belly. Mom was not amused at all. I guess she wasn't a visionary. I heard my dad relate this anecdote to his brothers a dozen times with increasing excitement, enthusiasm, and embellishment each time — but somehow the healing cloths, the dancing girls, and the band never materialized. Oh, well, I thought we were all going to be rich.

I've observed that patients who have a long-term relationship with a medical provider tend to develop affection for and trust in their doctor. The same was true for my dad. His patients loved and revered him. No doubt, some of that was due to his exceptional diagnostic capabilities, but mostly, I suspect, it was due in large part to the fact that his patients knew he loved them and respected them. They reciprocated that love and respect. **HE WAS A DEDICATED PHYSICIAN.**

If my dad had never gone to Laos and become a decorated veteran of the war in Southeast Asia, if he had not been a physician of repute, and an accomplished advocate for his community, if he had worked in obscurity in some other vocation, he would still be the greatest dad ever and a hero in the eyes of his children. **HE WAS A DEVOTED HUSBAND AND FATHER.**

My dad loved bird hunting, football, and especially Clemson football, but more than all of that combined, he loved America and serving his country in the military. A patriotic fervor ran deep in the core of his being. He loved that red, white, and blue flag and all that it stood for. **HE WAS A LOYAL AMERICAN.**

On laughter-silvered wings, he passed through our lives like a comet, swiftly, and all too briefly — and our lives were richer and fuller for having known him.

WHERE ARE THEY NOW?

Wife, Abbot — Mom taught school in Manning for a few more years, made a move or two, then married Ernest Carnes, the Associate Superintendent of Education for South Carolina, in 1986. They lived in Columbia, South Carolina, until his death. She continues to reside in Columbia.

Children —

Robert (Robin) — Family physician in Spartanburg, South Carolina, for forty years. Married to Carlotta Watson Jackson for forty years. They have nine children and fourteen grands.

Anne (Bristow) — Married to Walter Bristow, a gastroenterologist. Lives in Columbia, South Carolina. They have four children and five grands.

John Reed — Married to Kerri Mericle. Lives in Scottsdale, Arizona. Has two sons. Works for Tesla instructing potential buyers and new owners in the operation of Tesla electric vehicles. (The buyers love his slow, calm, reassuring southern drawl.)

Richard — Married to Laura Swearingen. Lives in Columbia, South Carolina. He works for a pharmaceutical company. They have two children. Richard calls on many physicians who still fondly remember our father.

Siblings —

Moultrie Richard (M.R., Robert's oldest brother) — Married to Pearl Smith. Had one daughter, Charlotte Ann. Married Hattie Plowden after Pearl's death. Worked for Savannah River Plant most of his working years.

Returned to Manning in later life. Deceased May 3, 1989.

Thomas "Jehu" — Married to Mary "Julia" Bradham, who died in a motor vehicle accident on November 8, 1968. Remarried to Katherine Hicklin a year later. Sheriff of Clarendon County from 1953-1981. Had one son, four daughters, and two stepsons. Deceased October 1, 1985.

William "Billy" Joseph — Married to Laura Gardner. Worked in farming in Clarendon County. Had two sons and one daughter. Deceased November 16, 1996.

Eunice Miriam — Married to Joseph "Buck" Norwood Epperson. Had four sons and one daughter. Worked as a teacher's assistant and a nurse's assistant. Deceased December 25, 2008.

Williford "Jimmy" Stuckey — Married Mary Nash. Had two sons and one daughter. Employed in school administration, principal of Edmund High School (now Sumter High School). Died suddenly at age forty-six on the day he was to defend his doctoral dissertation. Deceased April 3, 1968.

Edna Earl — Married Burney Lozano Hinson. Had one son and four daughters. Deceased October 14, 2000.

Ralph Singleton — Married Olivia McFadden. Had three daughters. Farmed in Clarendon County. Both Aunt Olivia and daughter Anna Lynn Floyd worked at Dad's office. Deceased January 4, 2018.

Scott Harmon — Married Roseanne Eadon. Had one son and three daughters. Was a Clarendon County farmer for more than fifty years, receiving numerous awards for achievements in soybean and corn production. Deceased March 20, 2011.

Carl Frank — Married Eleanor "Margaret" Durant. Had one son and one daughter. Farmed in Clarendon County. Deceased July 25, 2016.

Other —

Dr. Khammoung — No information available, which is not surprising since he was a high-profile Laotian physician/surgeon supporting the Communist resistance forces. We suspect that he became incognito when the Communists overran Laos, or, sad to say, he didn't make it out alive.

Vang Pao — Arrived in the United States in 1975 after Communists seized power in Laos. Had five wives, four he was forced to divorce upon entry into the United States. Reputed to have had twenty to thirty-two children. Beloved by his people, he continued to advocate for the Hmong people until his death January 6, 2011, in California.

Edgar "Pop" Buell — Secretly evacuated from Laos by dressing in a pilot's uniform, driven to the airport, and flown to Bangkok, Thailand. Lived in Bangkok the rest of his life. Died December 29, 1980, while visiting a friend in Manila, Philippines. Buried beside his wife, Mattie, in Edon Cemetery, Edon, Ohio.

Don Scott — Married to Nola for fifty-six years. Remarried after her death in 2014 to Doris Pearson. Served in Laos from 1964-1973. Remained in Vietnam working with World Vision until evacuated from Saigon in April 1975. Continued working for WV in Asia and Latin America. Returned to Canada in 1983, serving as President of World Vision Canada until 1996. Then returned to overseas work with WV until retirement in 2003. Currently lives on his wife's acreage in Wetaskiwin, Alberta, Canada.

Dr. Paul Sullivan — Retired from First Baptist Church of Manning after twenty-five years of ministry there, but continued to serve as interim pastor at four more churches. Married to Emily Kirby for fifty-six years. Died July 17, 2011, in Brunswick, Ga., near his children.

ACKNOWLEDGMENTS

Writing this book took me down memory lane with all of my first cousins — thirty-one in all — and their parents, my aunts and uncles. Our many family gatherings meant delicious, true-blue southern-fried food, laughing adults, and noisy children. My deepest affection and appreciation toward all of them for those special times and to those who shared their notes, quotes, and anecdotes about Dad — either recently or in documents collected over time. None of Dad's siblings were alive at the time of the writing of this book, but many recorded their memories after Dad's death, especially Aunt Eunice, and Uncles Ralph, Scott, Carl and Jehu. I had access to extensive letters by Uncle Jimmy, which I used to write about his time in World War II. Thanks to Cousin Bobby for passing these on to me. I owe a special thanks to my cousin Johanna Jones, one of the older cousins who actually grew up with Dad and who provided the most historical information. In addition to those who wrote their thoughts forty years ago, I want to say thank you to Cousins Anne Nivens, Charlotte Ann McCorquodale, Mike Epperson, and Beth Hinson Phillips for recently sharing their stories with me. I join my entire family in thanking our cousin Mike Epperson's wife, Doris, who compiled a Jackson and Singleton genealogy and history book for all of us. It provided or corroborated an abundance of information.

Thank you, Carter Jones, for the historical information regarding the founding of the Rescue Squad/EMS in Clarendon County and your recollections of "The Big Snow" in 1973. We all remember that one, don't we?

What a pleasure it was to talk with John Duffie and New York Yankee

Bobby Richardson, whose sharp memories added to the details about the American Legion Post 15 Sumter County baseball team. They fondly remembered playing baseball with Dad.

Although I tried to contact numerous people from Dad's time in Laos, I was able to connect with only one person that Dad talked about in his letters: Dr. Don Scott, the missionary with the Christian and Missionary Alliance. He was so gracious to respond to our first email, which led to other communication. In our phone conversation and emails, Dr. Scott affirmed so much of what Dad had to say about the conditions in Laos and the Laotians, as well as several particular personalities — including Pop Buell and Vang Pao, whom they both met. It meant so much to communicate with a spiritual leader in Dad's life during this difficult and life-threatening time, so I am especially thankful for the time he took to communicate with us and to send us some excellent pictures of life in Laos.

Numerous family friends wrote their stories about Dad a long time ago. This includes Dad's pastor and friend, who also spoke at his funeral — Dr. Paul Sullivan. Dr. Sullivan influenced my dad and me profoundly, so much so that one of my daughters named her first son after Dr. Sullivan because she has heard me talk about him so much. Other family friends included nurses at Clarendon Memorial Hospital, his own office staff and other medical personnel — Kermit Holliday, Anna Lynn Floyd (also a cousin), Pat Newman, Marie Mathis, and Asa Hatfield. I am grateful for their contributions decades ago, as well as to Kermit for recent conversations.

I greatly appreciate Dad's medical school classmates and/or medical associates who took time to write about their experiences with my father and then send them to my mom years ago. This includes Dr. J.J. Britton, Dr. Larry Heavrin, Dr. Peter Hairston, Dr. Vince Mosely, Dr. Robert Ridgeway, Dr. William Hunter, and Dr. Roger Gaddy. Dr. Mack Davis heard I was writing a book about my dad, so he called me up to tell me some of his favorite stories about him. What a fun conversation!

I am indebted as always to my readers who gave suggestions for writing a phrase or a paragraph a little differently — and to those who were willing to put their nose to the grindstone and look for the missing commas or the extra comma or the misspelled word or typo. One cannot have too many of these readers and people who just love grammar. These include my wife's college roommate, Cathy Parker, and her daughter, Lydia Parker, the youngest of ten and a linguistics major at the University of Florida; Brian Kiefer; our children; my siblings and mom; and Dr. Rudy Gray, the recently retired editor at Courier Publishing.

As always, I could not write any books without Carlotta, my lovely bride of forty years this very year. What am I saying? I probably would have no existence without her, because my life and our home truly revolve around her capable hands, her intelligent mind — but, most of all, her kind heart. She helped me in every phase of this and every book I've written — laboriously reading and typing from my longhand, doctor's handwriting! Yep, she deserves a medal, too, and maybe even hazardous duty pay! Thank you, my love!

My deepest affection and appreciation go to my brothers and sister — John Reed, Richard, and Anne — for, first of all, tolerating me as their oldest brother, and, secondly, for sharing their fond memories of our father. Although forty-three years have now come and gone since Dad's untimely passing, we remember him like it was yesterday and have missed him every day of our lives.

Of course, this book would not have been possible without the excellent record keeping of my mom. She saved many items from the journey she and my dad shared together. She even has his high school football jersey folded carefully in tissue paper, as well as his elementary school report cards. Prescient enough to know that a book about my dad would one day be written, she solicited letters from family and friends shortly after his death, which, as you saw, comprises a substantial portion of this book — and she organized them, including his letters from Laos, in such a way to make my job so much easier. When I surveyed the copious materials my mom had preserved, I realized anew that many people — patients, family, friends, and colleagues — really loved and appreciated Dr. Robert Jackson. I love you, Mom. I have an abiding respect for your persistent joyful demeanor. I dedicate Dad's book to you, for you deserve the honor.

Resources

3rd Armored Division (United States), https://en.wikipedia.org/wiki/3rd_
Armored_Division_(United_States). [accessed April 21, 2021].

Cates, Allen. "Air America." May 25, 2017. https://www.air-america.org/
air-america-history.html, [accessed June 20, 2021].

Clark, PhD, Sylvia H. *If These Walls Could Talk: Manning's Historic
Buildings.* Charleston, South Carolina: Evening Post Books, 2012.

Clark, PhD, Sylvia H. *Shadows of the Past: An Illustrated History of
Clarendon County, SC,* Clarendon County Historical Society. Virginia
Beach, Virginia: The Donning Company Publishers, 2005.

Cline, Lorrie. "I Met the Master Face to Face," English-Word Information:
Word Info About English Vocabulary. https://wordinfo.info/
unit/4493, [accessed March 7, 2022].

Duggan, Ervin, "Who's the True Patriot?" *The Washingtonian.*
Washington, DC: Washington Magazine, Inc., July 1980, Volume 15,
Number 10.

Fry, Charles W. "Lily of the Valley." Public domain.

Hamilton-Merritt, Jane. *Tragic Mountains: The Hmong, the Americans, and the Secret Wars for Laos, 1942-1992.* Bloomington and Indianapolis, Indiana: Indiana University Press, 1999.

Hinson, Mabel L. and Sylvia H. Clark, Marie M. Land, Lola W. Clark, Abbot L. Jackson. *Clarendon Cameos.* Manning: Clarendon County Historical Society. Limited Edition. 1976.

Ingram, PhD, Deborah and Jessica A. Montresor-Lopez, MPH, "Differences in Stroke Mortality Among Adults Aged 45 and Over: United States, 2010-2013, NCHS Data Brief No. 207," July 2015, National Center for Health Statistics, CDC, https://www.cdc.gov/nchs/products/databriefs/db207.html, [accessed July 12, 2021].

"International Voluntary Services," https://en.wikipedia.org/wiki/International_Voluntary_Services, [accessed April 21, 2021].

Jackson and Singleton Family: History and Genealogy. Compiled by Doris Epperson.

Leary, William M. "CIA Air Operations in Laos: 1954-1974," https://biotech.law.lsu.edu/cases/nat-sec/Vietnam/air-america.htm, April 14, 2007, [accessed April 21, 2021].

Magee, John Gillespie Jr. "High Flight." From Dr. Paul Sullivan's funeral notes. Public domain.

Makos, Adam. *Spearhead: An American Tank Gunner, His Enemy, and a Collision of Lives in World War II.* New York: Ballantine Books, 2019.

"Malaria," April 1, 2021, https://www.who.int/news-room/fact-sheets/detail/malaria, [accessed April 20, 2021].

Martin, Douglas. "General Vang Pao, Laotian Who Aided U.S., Dies at 81." *New York Times.* https://www.nytimes.com/2011/01/08/world/asia/08vangpao.html, [accessed July 12, 2021].

Miller, Kristie. *Ellen and Edith: Woodrow Wilson's First Ladies.* Lawrence, Kansas: University Press of Kansas, 2010.

"Parade Ends Concern Week," *The Sumter Daily Item*, May 8, 1971.

Paschal, Charles, Sports Editor, "Mantle Tried Hard to Hit Homer for Kids," *The Sumter Daily Item*, July 1, 1969, p. 8.

Pasculli, Len. "Bobby Richardson." *Society for American Baseball Research.* https://sabr.org/bioproj/person/bobby-richardson, updated October 31, 2020, [accessed March 13, 2021].

"Pop Buell, Hoosier at the Front," Internet Archive, March 7, 1965 episode of *The Twentieth Century* with Walter Cronkite. According to IMDB, the National Archives says it aired February 28, 1965, https://archive.org/details/The20thCPopHoosier, [accessed March 11, 2022].

"Pop Buell," https://en.wikipedia.org/wiki/Pop_Buell, [accessed April 21, 2021].

"South Carolina Fact Sheet." *American Heart Disease.* https://www.heart.org/-/media/files/about-us/policy-research/fact-sheets/quality-systems-of-care/quality-systems-of-care-south-carolina.pdf?la=en&hash, [accessed July 12, 2021].

Stewart, Drew. "Blizzard of '73 Frozen in Mind of Those Who Remember
    It Forty Years Later," WACH.comfox57, 1/8/2013, [accessed July 24,
    2021].

"The 3rd Armored Division During World War II." United States
    Holocaust Memorial Museum, https://encyclopedia.ushmm.org/
    content/en/article/the-3rd-armored-division, [accessed April 21, 2021].

" '52 Team Raps New F-15s." *The Sumter Daily Item*, July 1, 1969, p. 8.

Wilson, Edith Bolling. *My Memoir*. Indianapolis, Indiana: The Bobbs-
    Merrill Company, 1939.

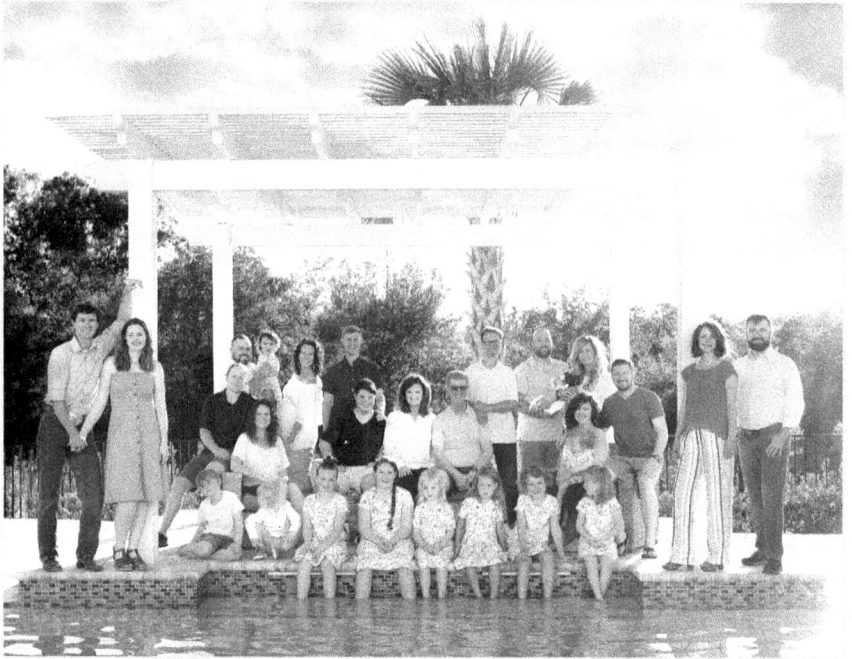

Dr. Jackson and his wife, Carlotta, their nine children, five sons-in-law, one daughter-in-law, and eleven grandchildren pictured above (six more grandchildren have been added since this photo from April 2021).

The Jacksons can be contacted for questions or for speaking engagements by visiting their website (https://www.jacksonfamilyministry.com), Facebook (Jackson Family Ministry) or Instagram (@jacksonfamilyministry). You can also hear them speak on a wide range of topics, but always through the lens of a biblical worldview, on their podcast entitled "More Than Medicine."

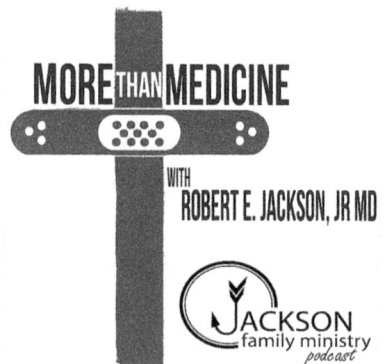

MORE THAN MEDICINE

WITH
ROBERT E. JACKSON, JR MD

JACKSON
family ministry
podcast

OTHER BOOKS BY DR. JACKSON

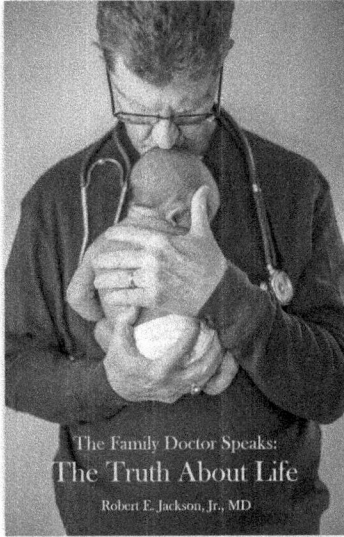

The Family Doctor Speaks:
The Truth About Life
(available at Amazon.com
and BarnesandNoble.com)

The Family Doctor Speaks:
The Truth About Life
Robert E. Jackson, Jr., MD

The Family Doctor Speaks:
The Truth About Seed Planting
(available at CourierPublishing.com,
Amazon.com, and BarnesandNoble.com)

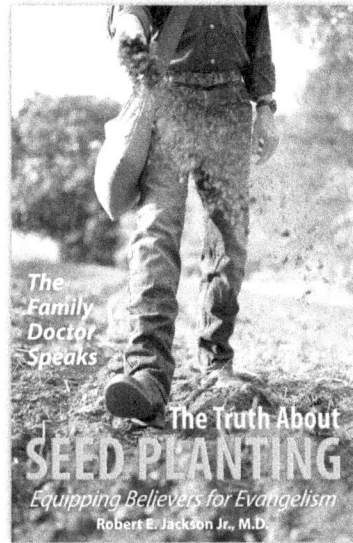

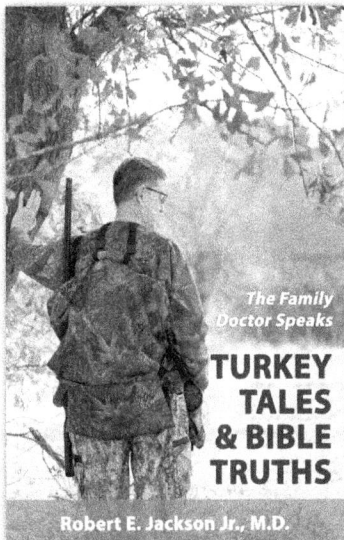

The
Family
Doctor
Speaks

The Truth About
SEED PLANTING
Equipping Believers for Evangelism
Robert E. Jackson Jr., M.D.

The Family
Doctor Speaks

TURKEY
TALES
& BIBLE
TRUTHS

Robert E. Jackson Jr., M.D.

The Family Doctor Speaks:
Turkey Tales & Bible Truths
(available at CourierPublishing.com,
Amazon.com, and BarnesandNoble.com)